Pitfalls in Ultrasound of Thyroid Nodules

Gaosong Wu • Qianqian Yuan
Rui Zhou

Pitfalls in Ultrasound of Thyroid Nodules

中国科学技术出版社
CHINA SCIENCE AND TECHNOLOGY PRESS
Springer

Gaosong Wu
Thyroid and Breast Surgery
Zhongnan Hospital of Wuhan University
Wuhan, China

Qianqian Yuan
Thyroid and Breast Surgery
Zhongnan Hospital of Wuhan University
Wuhan, China

Rui Zhou
Thyroid and Breast Surgery
Zhongnan Hospital of Wuhan University
Wuhan, China

ISBN 978-981-19-8872-1 ISBN 978-981-19-8873-8 (eBook)
https://doi.org/10.1007/978-981-19-8873-8

Jointly published with China Science and Technology Press
The print edition is not for sale in China (Mainland). Customers from China (Mainland) please order the print book from: China Science and Technology Press.

This Springer imprint is published by the registered company Springer Nature Singapore Pte Ltd.
The registered company address is: 152 Beach Road, #21-01/04 Gateway East, Singapore 189721, Singapore

Synopsis

From the perspective of surgeons, more than 50 cases diagnosed with clinically common typical thyroid nodules were specially selected. Common misdiagnosed cases and part of difficult cases in the ultrasound diagnosis of thyroid nodules were covered. Each case was systematically introduced as follows: clinical data, ultrasound data, ultrasound evaluation preoperatively, gross specimen and pathological diagnosis, discussion: pitfalls and causes analyses. Thyroid nodules were deeply multi-dimensional interpreted by means of ultrasound images and video, specimen dissection and pathological examination, the causes of misdiagnoses were analyzed as well. This book was written uniquely with great practicability and multiple pictures, which had guiding significance for thyroid surgeons and ultrasound experts.

Premise

Thyroid is a superficial glandular tissue with uniform texture; ultrasound is the preferred method of examination for thyroid disease. Detecting thyroid nodules by ultrasound is very sensitive; 2–3 mm thyroid nodules can be detected. The detection rate of thyroid nodules is 19–68%; 7–15% were malignant. The detection rate of unpalpable thyroid nodules is 50–60% in persons more than 60 years old. The main purpose of ultrasound diagnosis is to distinguish benign and malignant nodules. Under the guidance of ultrasound, fine needle aspiration cytology can be performed for thyroid nodules with malignant signs, avoiding over treatment for benign thyroid nodules, saving precious medical resources, and avoiding morbidity. Ultrasonography is an important tool for thyroid surgeons in the diagnosis and treatment of thyroid nodules, playing an important role in assisting preoperative diagnosis and treatment. A suitable ultrasound diagnosis book helps surgeons to better carry out clinical work, making up for the lack of knowledge in anatomy and clinical pathology for ultrasound imaging physicians. Thyroid nodules can be diagnosed by dynamic ultrasound images of different sections collected by surgeons, requiring a relatively high level of skills of the sonographer. Misdiagnosis of thyroid nodules might occur owing to the evaluation by different physicians and instrument utilization. Benign nodules might be misdiagnosed as malignant nodules to be overtreated, or the malignant nodules might be missed or underdiagnosed.

This is the first book which has systematically summarized the ultrasound thyroid nodules from the perspective of surgeons, closely combining the imaging and clinical characteristics. During the clinical practice in our country, effective contact and communication lack between ultrasound imaging physician, pathology physician and surgeons. The surgeons act as a bridge, asking history preoperatively, combined with ultrasound diagnosis, observing the texture of nodules intraoperatively, confirming the ultrasound diagnosis by pathological examination postoperatively. Preoperative ultrasound evaluation can be detected by surgeons to decrease the missed and misdiagnosed nodules, improving the coincidence rate of ultrasound and pathological diagnosis. Department of Thyroid and Breast Surgery in Wuhan University Zhongnan Hospital accumulated multiple experience in the diagnosis of malignant thyroid nodules. This book contains abundant clinical cases and can be used as a teaching book for beginner and an expert-led training course.

Thanks for the assistance of Jinxuan Hou, Jiuyang Liu, Qianqian Yuan, Lewei Zheng during the book editing.

Wuhan University Zhongnan Hospital
Wuhan, China

Gaosong Wu

Contents

Misdiagnosis of Thyroid Nodule Calcification

1

Compared with CT and MRI, ultrasound can provide detailed information and high efficiency for diagnosis. As an easy to use, affordable, noninvasive, nonradioactive, and repeatable instrument, ultrasound has been the preferred method to diagnose thyroid nodules (Fig. 1.1). Calcification in the thyroid nodules is quite common, which is an important sonographic finding. Calcification can occur in benign and malignant nodules. Size, quantity, shape, and distribution of the calcification in the diagnosis and differential diagnosis of malignant nodules are still controversial.

According to the findings of ultrasound imaging, calcification can be classified into four types: a. large calcification: hyperechogenicity with acoustic shadowing and punctate, arcs, or other irregularities hyperechogenicity >1 mm in diameter and may occur in both benign and malignant lesions (Figs. 1.2, 1.3, and 1.4); b. microcalcification: psammomatous, needle-like, granules, and punctate calcification <1 mm (Fig. 1.5); c. peripheral calcification: large calcifications around the thyroid nodules, present as peripheral curved or eggshell-like calcifications; and d. isolated calcification: A single coarse calcification <5 mm without tumor tissue around.

Calcifications exist in different histologic types of thyroid tumors, including papillary, medullary, and anaplastic tumors. Histologically, thyroid calcification is divided into psammomatous and malnutrition calcification. Pathologists describe sand granule as concentric circles of calcified small bodies (8th edition of Pathology edited by Li Yulin), one of the characteristic findings of papillary thyroid carcinoma, composed of laminated basophilic spherical concretions, which can be manifested as punctate hyperechogenic foci in ultrasound (Fig. 1.6). Among the types of calcifications, microcalcification is the most specific for the diagnosis of papillary thyroid carcinoma. In a retrospective study of 1498 surgically treated thyroid nodules, the detection rate of calcification in malignant nodules by preoperative ultrasound was 49.6%, while benign nodules was 15.7%. The detection rate of microcalcification in malignant nodules was significantly more than that of benign nodules. The sensitivity and specificity of microcalcification in the diagnosis of malignant thyroid nodules were 33.7% and 93.6%, respectively.

Hyperechoic foci is the local lesion that presents significantly increased echogenicity than the surrounding tissues, which varies in size, shape, and distributed in single or cluster, or with acoustic shadowing behind. Microcalcification is punctate hyperechogenicity, while punctate hyperechogenicity may not be the calcification. Microcalcification may present as colloid crystallography, fibrotic, or intracapsular hemorrhage on ultrasound. For example, some ultrasound images present irregularly distributed microscopic, small

Supplementary Information The online version contains supplementary material available at https://doi.org/10.1007/978-981-19-8873-8_1.

G. Wu et al., *Pitfalls in Ultrasound of Thyroid Nodules*,
https://doi.org/10.1007/978-981-19-8873-8_1

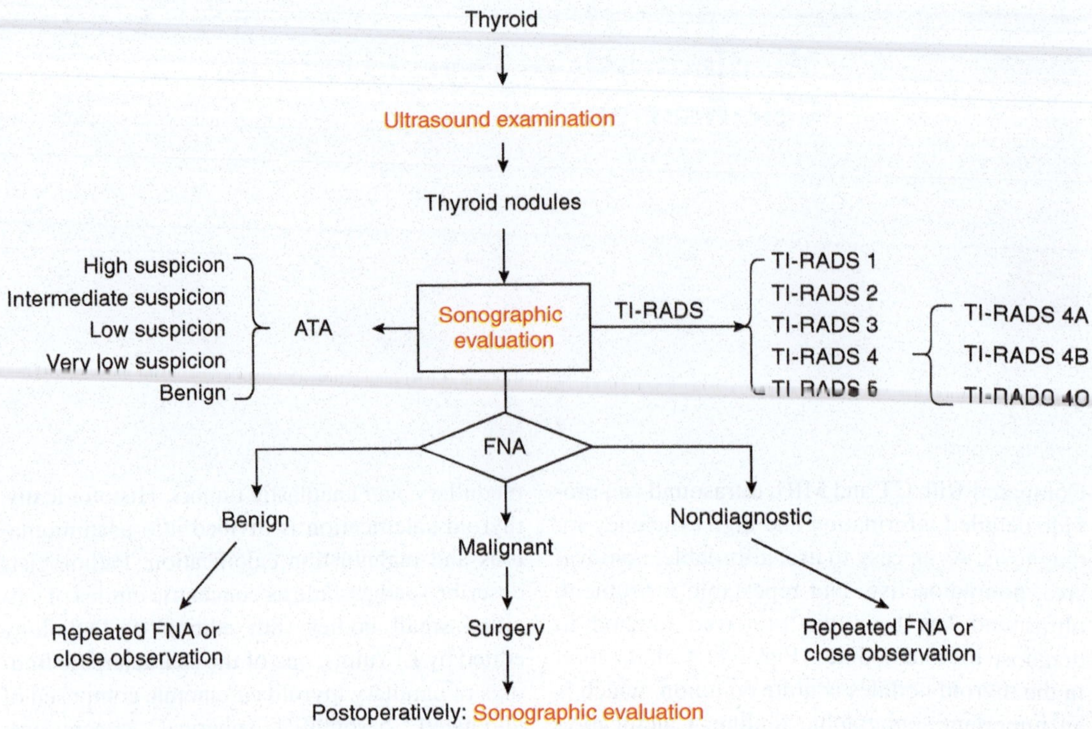

Fig. 1.1 Algorithm for evaluation and management of patients with thyroid nodules based on TI-RADS and ATA pattern and FNA cytology. US: ultrasound, ATA: American Thyroid Association, TI-RADS: Thyroid Imaging Reporting and Data System

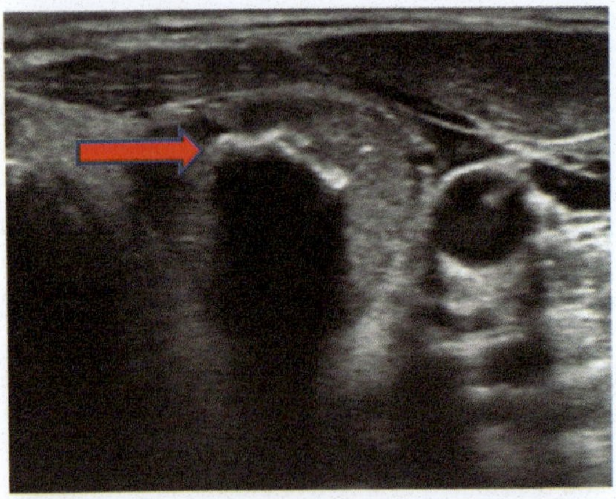

Fig. 1.2 Arc coarse calcification. A 50-year-old male patient, a hypoechoic 4.6 cm × 2.0 cm nodule in the left lobe with clear margin with arc coarse calcification. Diagnosis: nontoxic nodular thyroid goiter concomitant with adenomatous nodule

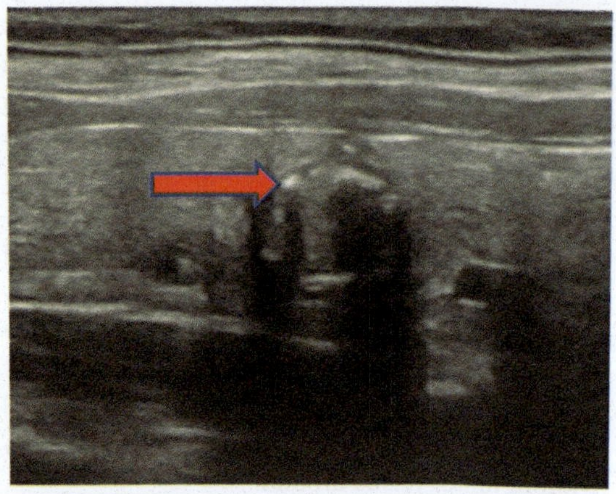

Fig. 1.3 Punctate coarse calcification. A 35-year-old male patient, a hypoechoic 1.9 cm × 1.2 cm nodule in the left lobe with an ill-defined margin with several coarse calcifications. Diagnosis: thyroid papillary carcinoma

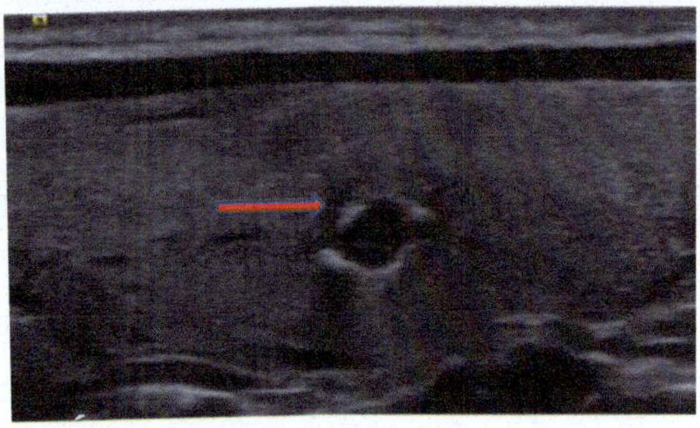

Fig. 1.4 Peripheral calcification. A 37-year-old male patient, a hypoechoic 0.5 cm nodule in the left lobe with surrounding ring hyperechoic foci. Diagnosis: thyroid papillary microcarcinoma

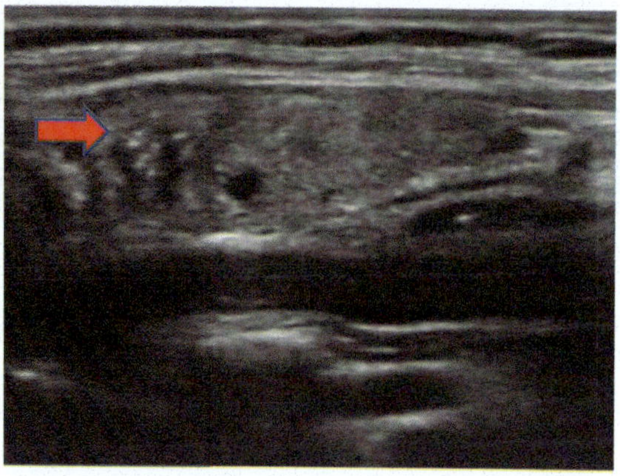

Fig. 1.5 Needle-like calcification. A 34-year-old female patient, a hypoechoic 0.9 cm nodule in the left lobe with punctate hyperechoic foci. Diagnosis: thyroid papillary carcinoma

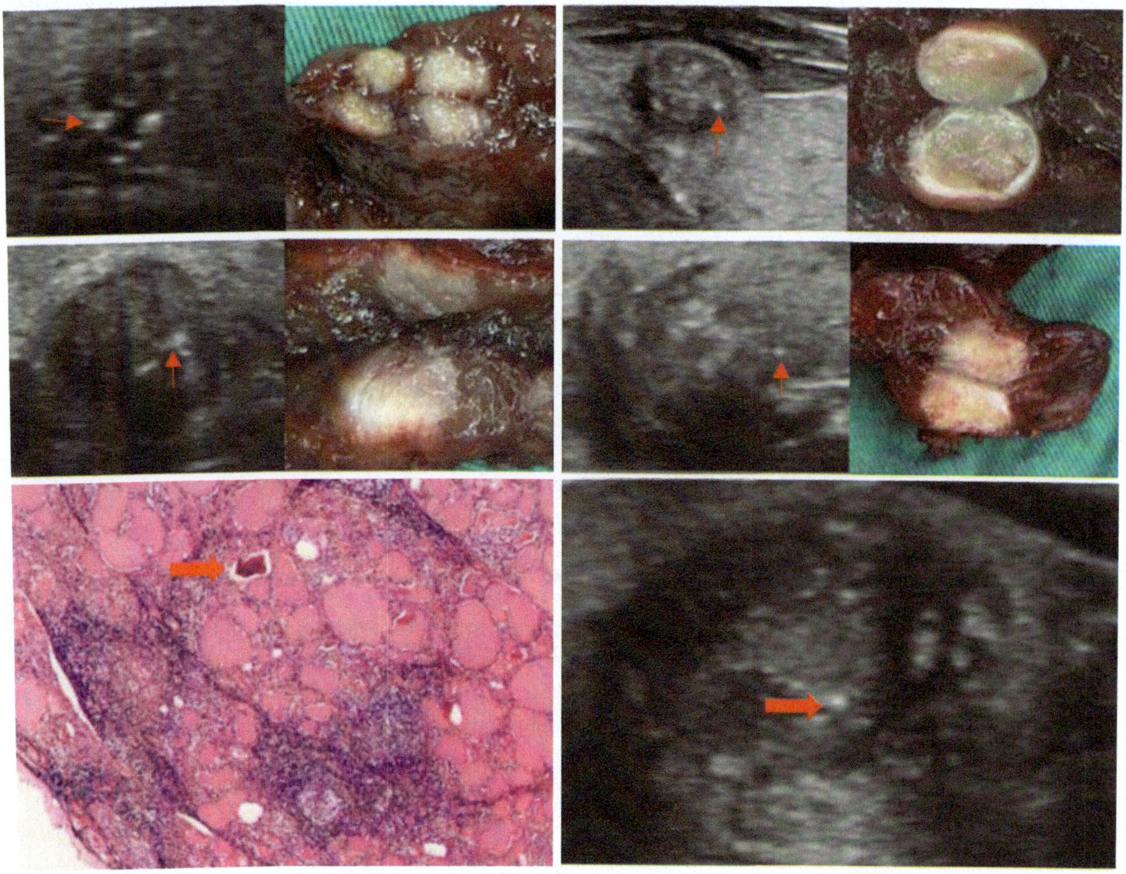

Fig. 1.6 The red arrow indicates the sand granule in which microcalcification is observed histologically (hematoxylin and eosin stain, X100)

punctate hyperechogenicity, sections were fibrous tissue at low magnification accordingly and were calcium salt deposition distributed in hyperplastic fibrous tissue at high magnification. Some ultrasound images present small punctate hyperechogenicity, sections show the bands of fibrous tissue at low magnification accordingly, and no calcification occurred at high magnification. Therefore, the punctate hyperechogenicity on the ultrasound imaging is not exactly equivalent to the sand granule diagnosed by pathology.

Case 1

Clinical information: A 60-year-old female patient presented with a cervical nodules for more than 2 months with normal thyroid function and without clinical signs.

Ultrasonic information: Ultrasound report is the first information while the picture is not clear owing to the natural quality of printed paper. Hence, the clinician obtains the information mainly through the ultrasound description. The following ultrasound report indicated hypoechogenic lesion with punctate hyperechogenicity foci and color blood flow on the left lobe, which was classified as TI-RADS 4b (Fig. 1.7). Nodules can be palpated on this patient, and fine needle aspiration cytology was recommended. This patient preferred surgery owing to anxiety about the disease after patient education.

Preoperative ultrasound evaluation: In order to provide a better treatment plan, the thyroid ultrasound was reevaluated (Fig. 1.8).

Gross specimen and pathological diagnosis: Figs. 1.9 and 1.10.

Discussion: Misdiagnosis analysis and prevention strategies

1. *Misdiagnosis analysis of hyperechogenicity in nodular goiters*
   Relatively insufficient thyroid hormones stimulate the pituitary gland secreting increased thyroid-stimulating hormone (TSH). Thyroid gland tissue appears uneven hyperplasia and then forms nodules under the long-term stimulation of higher levels of TSH. Tissues around the nodules are often have wrapped by an obvious fibrous tissue.

Sonographic findings

Thyroid scan:

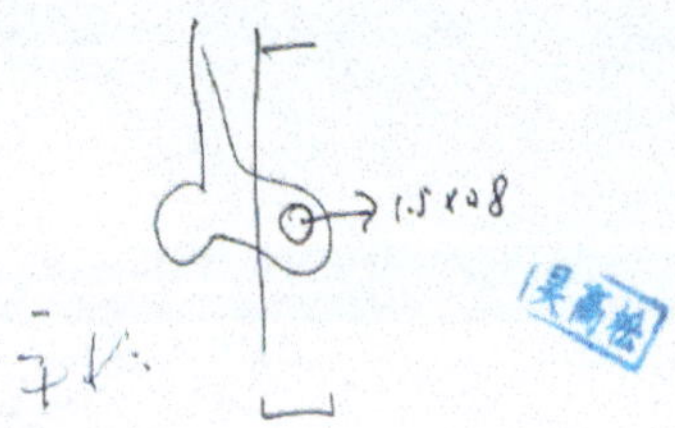

Left lobe: 4.1 cm × 1.5 cm × 1.2 cm;

Right lobe: 3.7cm× 1.6cm× 1.2cm;

Anteroposterior diameter of thyroid isthmus: 0.20 cm;

The shape was normal on the transverse view, the echogenicity of parenchyma are uneven.

A 1.5 cm × 0 .8cm hypoechogenic foci was visible in the left lobe, the margin was not clear, and the echogenicity inside was uneven, with punctate hyperechogenicity inside, and the color blood flow signal was detected. Several hypoechogenic and anechoic areas were visible in the bilateral lobes, with clear margin and uneven echogenicity, one of is 0.2 cm× 0.2 cm in size without obvious color blood flow signal.

Sonographic indicates:

Hypoechogenic nodules with calcification in the left lobe (TI-RADS 4b)

Hypoechogenic or anechoic lesions in the bilateral lobes (TI-RADS 3)

Fig. 1.7 Sonographic report of Case 1

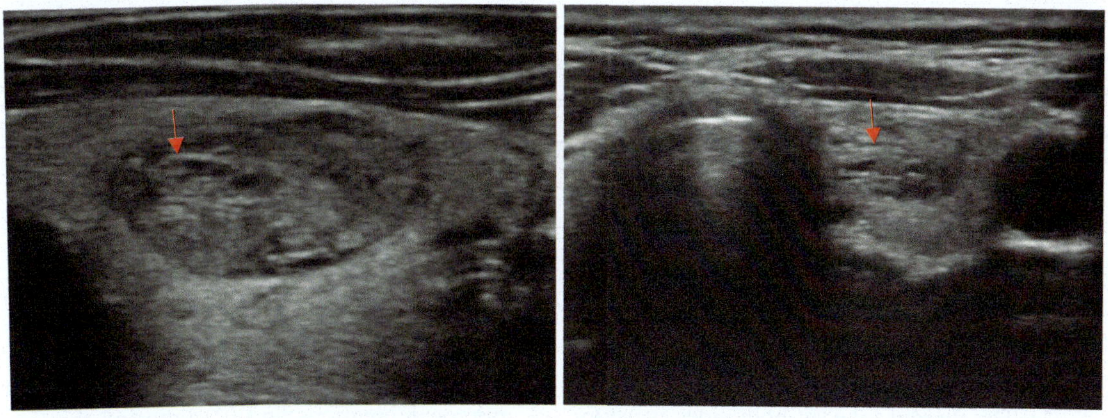

Fig. 1.8 Preoperative ultrasound evaluation for case 1. Hypoechoic nodule was detected on left lobe, scattered streaked hyperechogenicity was seen between hypoechoic nodules. Rotate the probe in different directions, linear hyperechogenicity could be detected composed of punctate hyperechogenicity (red arrows). Scattered linear echogenicity formed by fibrous tissue hyperplasia could be detected between nodular thyroid goiter, showing punctate hyperechogenicity on transverse view in ultrasound. The probe should be rotated in different directions in order to misdiagnose the streaked hyperechogenicity as a punctate calcification

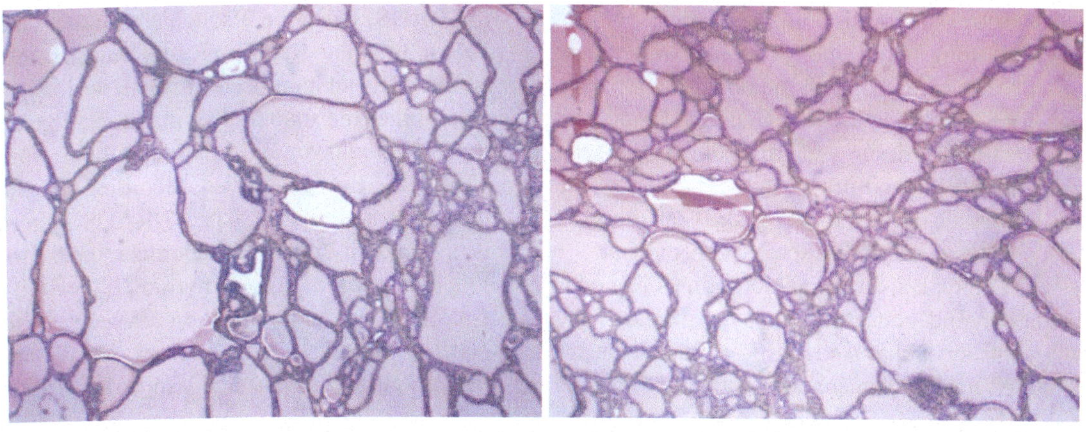

Fig. 1.9 Pathological diagnosis: (left) nodular thyroid goiter

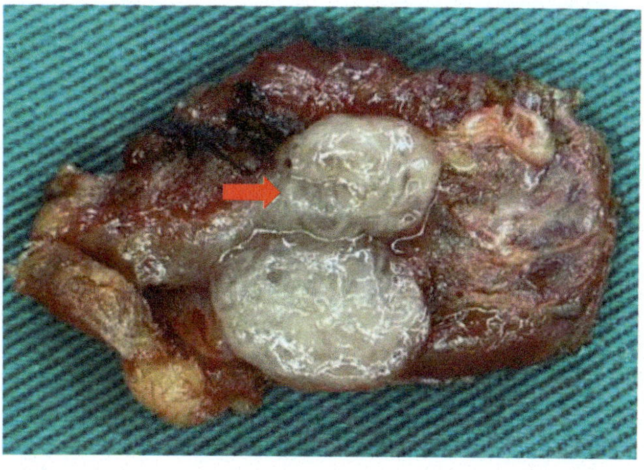

Fig. 1.10 Gross specimen. A tough nodule could be palpated in the specimen. A canous 0.5 cm nodule with a clear margin was seen after resecting the gland along the longest diameter of the nodule. The incision is effortless. Follicles of varying sizes can be seen in the microscopic thyroid, and no abnormal type of cells. Pathological diagnosis: (left) nodular thyroid goiter

The compression of the inside and surrounding interstitial blood vessels lead to insufficient blood supply to the nodules, further secondary changes to the nodules, bleeding, necrosis, fibrosis, and cystic degeneration. Some nodular thyroid goiters exist hemosiderin, cholesterol deposition, and calcification inside. Therefore, the ultrasound manifestations of nodular thyroid goiter are diverse and difficult to distinguish.

Common ultrasound manifestations of nodular goiter are as follows:

(1) The thyroid lobe on both sides is asymmetrically enlarged.
(2) Multiple nodules and unevenly distributed.
(3) The echogenicities are diverse, showing hypoechogenicity, hyperechogenicity, or sightly hyperechogenicity. Nodules can be cystic, cystic solid, and solid.
(4) Strong hyperechoic foci and liquid dark areas are visible in the nodule.
(5) Scattered linear echogenicity formed by fibrous tissue hyperplasia can be seen between nodules.
(6) Cystic degeneration, eggshell calcification, or coarse calcification are concomitant.

The typical sonographic findings of nodular thyroid goiter present hyperplasia as the mainstay and mixed cystic-solid, and scattered linear echogenicities formed by fibrous dimensional tissue hyperplasia can be seen between the nodules (Figs. 1.11 and 1.12).

Scattered linear echogenicities formed by fibrous dimensional tissue hyperplasia are easily misdiagnosed as punctate calcifications, requiring a multidirectional change of the probe; multiple cystic regions are visible on longitudinal section, separated by a delicate diaphragm, and are honeycomb-shaped, presenting as a manifestation of nodular goiter. Reasons for misdiagnoses are: (1) treating the punctate hyperechogenicity as microcalcifications and (2) ignoring the fine linear echogenicity in the nodules, which are the characteristic of nodular thyroid goiter (Fig. 1.13).

2. *Confusion about TI-RADS classification*
In 2009, Horvath et al. first proposed the Thyroid Imaging Reporting and Data System (TI-RADS) based on a scheme similar to the Breast Imaging Reporting and Data System (BI-RADS) lexicon used in breast lesions. It recombines the sonographic manifestations of thyroid nodules and divides them into TI-RADS 1–6 categories according to the degree of malignancy. The TI-RADS system is a standard tool to standardize the sonographic terminology of thyroid. It not only simplifies the communication between physicians and patients, and between physicians, but also allows the research standards between

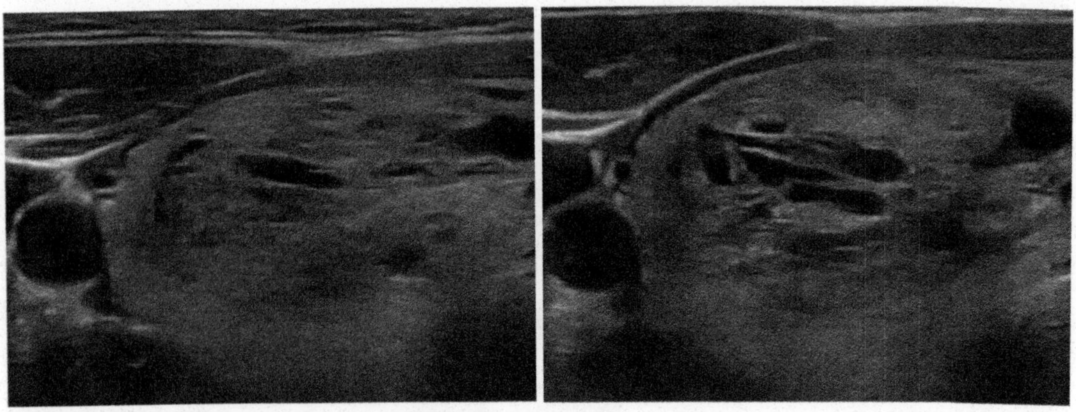

Fig. 1.11 Typical ultrasonic imaging of nodular thyroid goiter. 2D: A 4 cm × 2 cm × 3.2 cm mixed echoic foci with a clear margin and streaked sightly hyperechogenicity

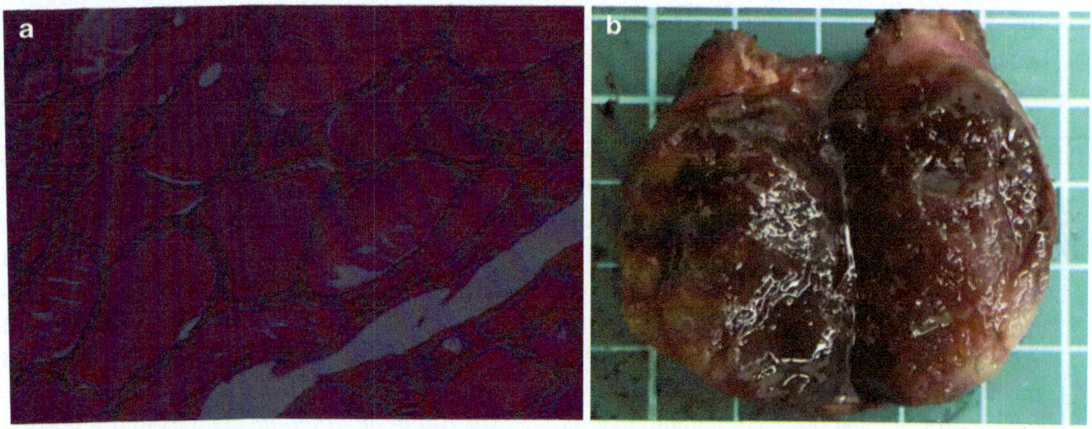

Fig. 1.12 Typical pathology and gross of nodular thyroid goiter. A Under microscope: thyroid tissue hyperplasia, composed of follicles of varying sizes, filled with colloid and normal cells. B Gross specimen: 4 cm Gray-red tissue with a soft texture

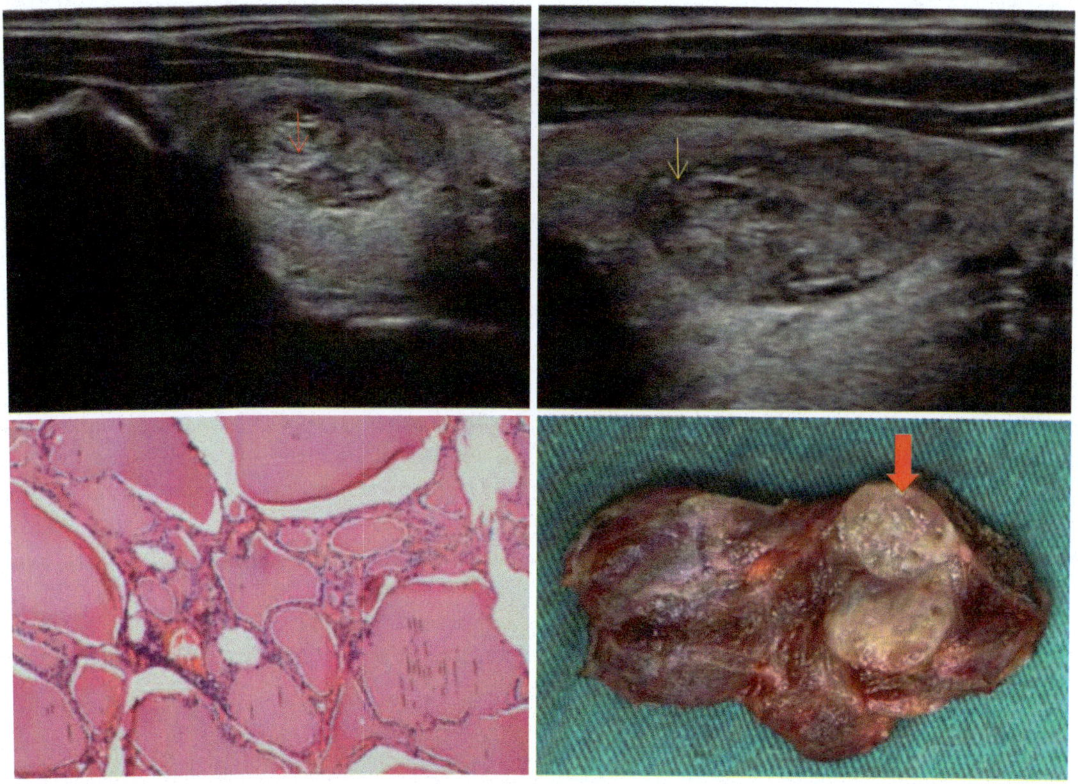

Fig. 1.13 Sporadic linear echogenicity formed by fibrous tissue hyperplasia between nodules is easily misdiagnosed as punctate calcification (pathological diagnosis: nodular thyroid goiter)

different medical institutions to be unified. Ultrasound indicates the first information when patients were admitted. TI-RADS is stratified into 1–5 categories, and the frequency of malignancy for each category was estimated: 0% for TI-RADS 1 and 2, <5% for TI-RADS 3, 5% to 10% for TI-RADS 4A, 10% to 80% for TI-RADS 4B, and >80% for TI-RADS 5. Ultrasound signs of malignant thyroid nodules include parenchyma hypoechogenicity, or extreme hypoechogenicity, differential lobe or ill-defined margin, microcalcification, and nodule that is taller than wide. Once aforementioned malignant signs are presented, the nodule can be classified as 4, with only one malignant sign being 4a, two signs being 4b, three and four signs being 4c, and having more than four signs being classified as 5 (Table 1.1).

Experienced clinicians can evaluate composition, echogenicity, margin, calcification, and shape of the nodule according to the sonographic findings. Hypoechogenicity, unclear margin, microcalcification, nodule that is taller than wide, and increased nodular vascularity are suspected of carcinoma. 2017 ACR TI-RADS Grading Standards (composition, echogenicity, shape, margin, echogenic foci) are the same as usual Thyroid nodules are evaluated in a benign and malignant manner. In practice, TI-RADS classification is very subjective. It is impossible to score each nodule according to the accurate ACR TI-RADS Grading Standards. The same patient in different hospitals, or different physicians in the same hospital may show different TI-RADS classifications. Hence, once get the ultrasound reports, in addition to looking at the classification in the description, they must also have a certain judgment ability, clinician should evaluate the size and shape of the nodule, in addition to the TI-RADS classification.

Case 2

Clinical information: A 37-year-old male patient presented without symptoms. T3, T4, and TSH levels were normal. Specialized physical examination: A tough nodule about 1.5 cm in the left thyroid lobe could be palpated, which moves up and down along with swallowing.

Ultrasonic information: Ultrasound reporting is relatively simple. TI-RADS classification has not been present. Sonographic description: mixed echogenicity nodules, ill-defined margin. Sonographic information is insufficient. clear. Fine needle aspiration cytology was recommended for this patient.

Preoperative ultrasound evaluation: Fig. 1.14

Preoperative ultrasonic reevaluation of the thyroid (Fig. 1.15)

Site: nodule detected in the middle of the left lobe

Size: 1.9 cm * 1.6 cm

Composition: main solid

Echogenicity: hypoechogenicity

Margin: ill-defined margin

Hyperechic lesion: Focal punctate hyperechogenicity

Total score: 7, ACR TI-RADS 5, highly suspected as malignant.

Gross specimen and pathological diagnosis: Fig. 1.16

Discussion: Misdiagnosis analysis and prevention strategies

Microcalcification refers to pinnacle-like or punctate hyperechogenicity, often clustered into

Table 1.1 Kwak TI-RADS

Suspicious ultrasound features	Classification	Suspicious features	Probability carcinoma (%)
Solid component	1	0	0
Hypoechogenicity or marked hypoechogenicity	2	0	0
Microlobulated or irregular margin	3	0	1.7
Microcalcification	4a	1	3.3
	4b	2	9.2
	4c	3~4	44.4~72.4
Taller-than-wide shape	5	5	87.5

Sonographic findings

Right lobe: Transverse diameter is 17 mm, anteroposterior diameter is 17 mm.

Left lobe: Transverse diameter is 16 mm, anteroposterior diameter is 19 mm.

Isthmus: anteroposterior diameter is 25 mm.

Size and shape of the thyroid gland is acceptable. Left lobe is sightly larger, and the capsule is in integrity. A 19.4 cm×16.5cm nodule with mixed echogenicity and ill-defined margin was detected in the left lobe. CDFI: Colored blood flow signals were detected.

Sonographic indicates

Nodule with mixed echogenicity in left lobe, nodular thyroid goiter?

Fig. 1.14 Sonographic report of Case 2

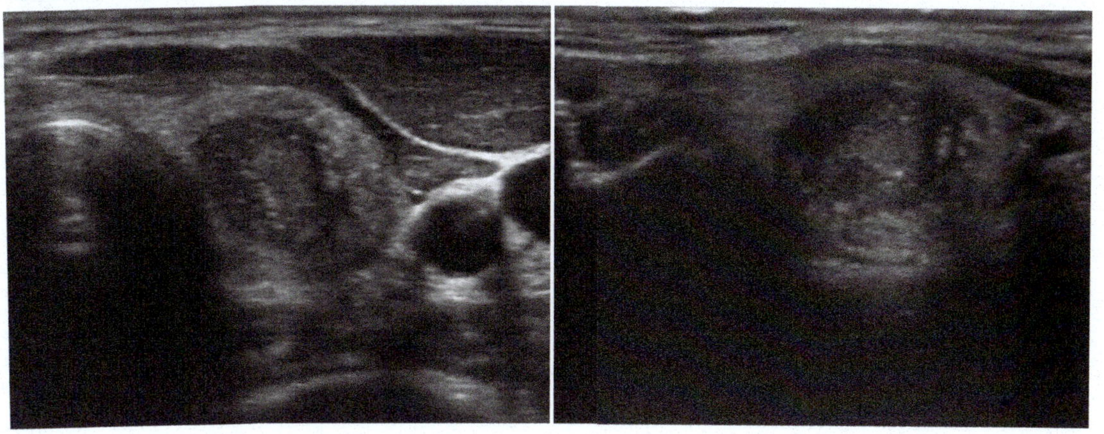

Fig. 1.15 Preoperative ultrasonic reevaluation. A 37-year-old female patient detected a thyroid nodule while routine examination. Preoperative ultrasonic reevaluation of the thyroid was performed, and classify the nodule according to the updated ACR TI-RADS category

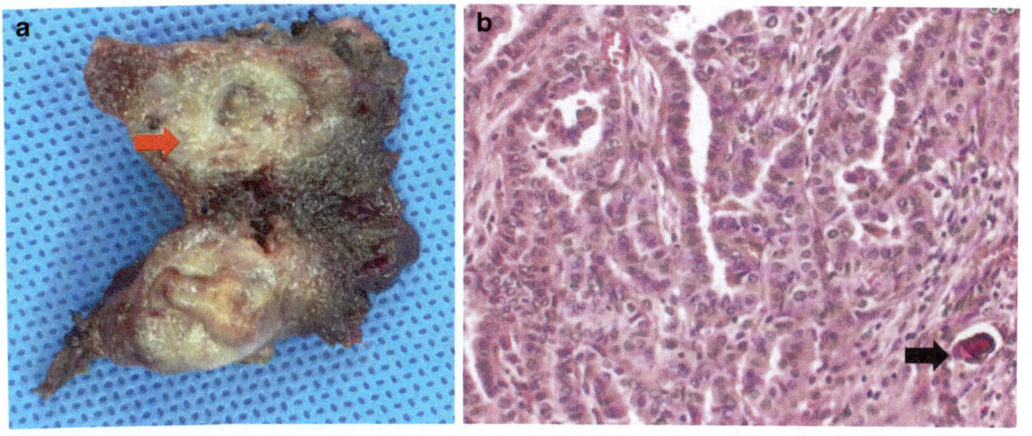

Fig. 1.16 Gross specimen and pathological diagnosis of case 2. (**a**) The texture of nodule is hard and adhesive to the surrounding muscles with frosted incision feeling. (**b**) Under microscope: sand granule (red arrow). A 1.9 cm × 1.5 cm gray-yellow-gray-white lesion could be seen, not clearly demarcated from surrounding tissues (black arrow). Pathological diagnosis: (left) papillary thyroid carcinoma

clusters without acoustic shadowing behind. Microcalcification is basically equivalent to sand granules pathologically, which is a characteristic manifestation of malignant nodules. The sand granule observed pathologically is a 50–70 μm calcium phosphate structure. This calcium phosphate often manifests as a layered concentric circle structure distributed in multiple fine granules.

Solitary hypoechoic nodule with small hyperechoic foci is the ultrasonic feature for papillary thyroid carcinoma, showing small punctate hyperechogenicity, clear margin, without acoustic shadowing, present as sand granules pathologically. The ultrasound of nodular thyroid goiter shows "punctate calcification foci," with an ill-defined margin and a comet-tail sign. The infiltration of lymphocytes formed the nodule. Increased thyroid follicles around the nodules and close colloid inside promote acoustic penetration, resulting in multiple reflections behind the lymphocyte nodules, showing a comet-tail sign, which is different from the microcalcification in thyroid carcinoma (Figs. 1.17 and 1.18).

Case 3

Clinical information: A 41-year-old male patient presented with cervical mass. T3, T4, and TSH levels were normal. Specialized physical examination: A tough nodule about 2.0*1.5 cm in the left thyroid lobe could be palpated, which moves up and down along with swallowing.

Ultrasonic information: Sonographic reports in different hospitals have controversy on the isoechoic or hypoechoic nodule. Hypoechoic nodules increased the probability of malignancy (Figs. 1.19 and 1.20).

Preoperative ultrasound evaluation: Nodule and surrounding gland present the same echogenicity. Fine needle aspiration cytology was recommended for this patient. This patient was required to receive surgery owing to neck discomfort (Fig. 1.21).

Gross specimen and pathological diagnosis: Figs. 1.22 and 1.23

Discussion: Misdiagnosis analysis and prevention strategies

Thyroid tumor The composition of cells and interstitium in thyroid tumor, cell differentiation degree, cyst formation, hemorrhage, necrosis, and fibrosis in interstitium are the basis of ultrasonic image. If the nodules were accompanied by hemorrhage, necrosis, uneven distribution of fibrous tissue, vascular hyperplasia, or inflammatory cell infiltration in the interstitium, uneven echogenicity was present on the ultrasonic image.

Nodular thyroid goiter is common in benign thyroid tumors, characterized by the formation of variable follicles pathologically. The follicles contain jelly-like substances and form a cyst cav-

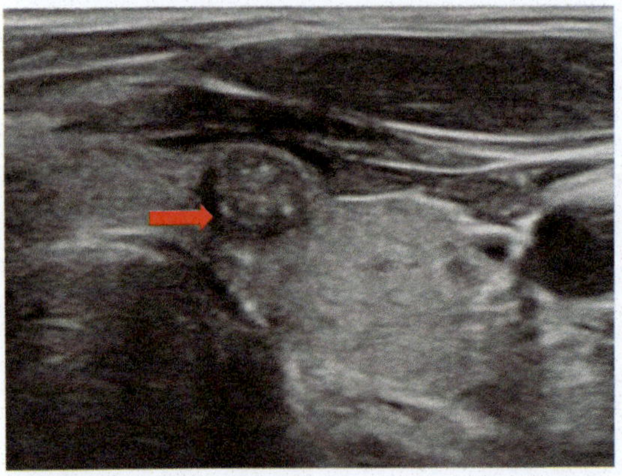

Fig. 1.17 Microcalcification. A 46-year-old male patient with a 1.0 cm × 0.9 cm hypoechoic nodule with punctate hyperechoic foci in the left lobe. Diagnosis: thyroid papillary carcinoma

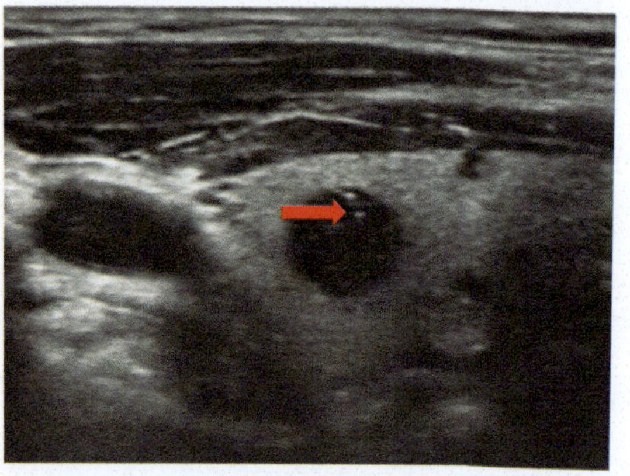

Fig. 1.18 Microcalcification. A 63-year-old male patient with a 1.0 cm × 1.9 cm hypoechoic nodule with punctate hyperechoic foci in the left lobe. Diagnosis: thyroid papillary carcinoma. A comet-tail sign (red arrow)

Sonographic findings:

Thyroid scan:

The shape and size were normal on the transverse view, the echogenicity of parenchyma are uniform. A 5.8 mm* 3.5 mm hypoechoic regular margin nodule was detected in the middle of the left lobe. A 24.0 mm* 12.6 mm isoechoic nodule was detected in the upper middle of the right lobe, with hypoechoic halo and a small patchy anechoic area and a punctate hyperechogenic foci are seen inside.

CDFI: The hypoechoic nodule on left lobe showed blood flow signal, the isoechoic nodule on right lobe showed ring blood flow signal.

Sonographic indicates:

Multiple thyroid nodules (solid, cystic). Isoechoic solid nodule in the upper middle of the right lobe was concomitant with multiple calcifications, and further examination is recommended.

Fig. 1.19 Sonographic report of Case 3.1

Sonographic findings

Right lobe: 5.8 cm × 1.9 cm × 1.7 cm.

Left lobe: 4.1 cm × 1.5 cm × 1.2 cm.

Isthmus: anteroposterior diameter is 0.17 cm.

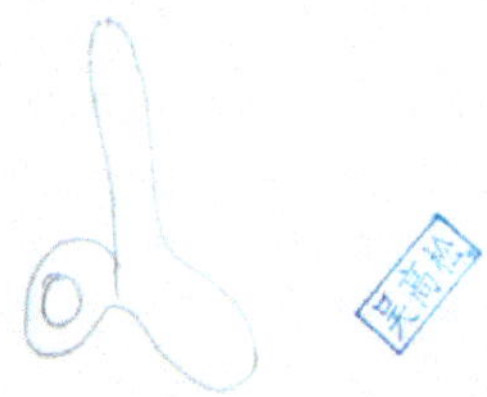

The shape and size were normal on the transverse view, the echogenicity of parenchyma are uniform. A 0.6 cm × 0.4 cm hypoechoic regular margin nodule was detected in the middle of the left lobe, with uniform echogenicity, blood flow, a small patchy anechoic area and hypoechogenic foci inside. A 0.3 cm × 0.2 cm enlargement and a small punctate hyperechogenicity with blood flow were detected inside. Multiple hypo- and anechoic areas with ill-defined margin were detected, one of which is a 0.2 cm × 0.2 cm punctate hyperechogenicity without blood flow.

Sonographic indicates:

Hypoechoic nodules on the left thyroid lobe with calcification (TI-RADS 4a)

Hypoechoic nodules on the left thyroid lobe (TI-RADS 3)

Hypo- and anechoic areas on the bilateral thyroid gland (colloid cysts).

Fig. 1.20 Sonographic report of Case 3.2

ity. Small nipples by follicular epithelial cells overproliferated, less interstitial components, and the large difference in acoustic resistance between the colloid and follicular epithelium formed multi-interface reflections. Therefore, hyperechogenicity and liquid anechoic area are often detected. Papillary tumor is more common in thyroid carcinoma, with large and overlapping cancer cells, few interstitial components, and no reflex interface formed in ultrasonic images, so solid hypoechogenicity is often detected.

If there is bleeding or cystic degeneration of the nodule, ultrasound shows a cystic-solid or cystic mixture of masses. Nodular thyroid goi-

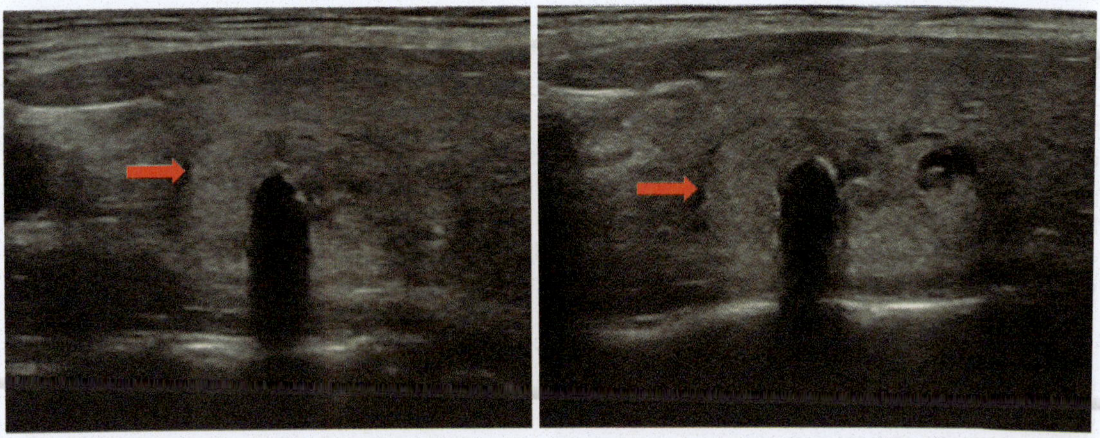

Fig. 1.21 Preoperative ultrasonic reevaluation. 2D: A 24.2 mm × 14.6 mm isoechoic nodule could be detected in the right lobe with surrounding hypoechoic areola, in which sheet anechoic area, a 0.3 cm × 0.2 cm coarse punctate hyperechogenicity and small punctate hyperechogenicity were detected

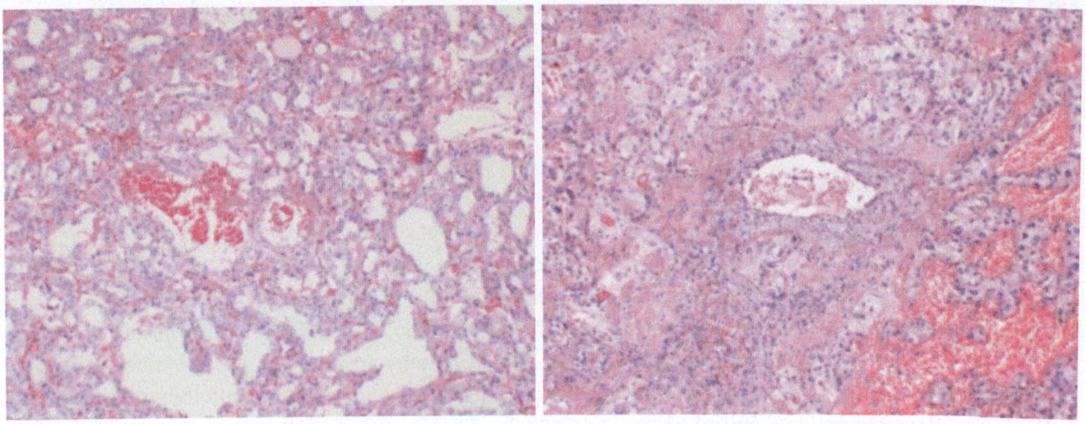

Fig. 1.22 Pathological diagnosis of case 3. (Right lobe) Nodular thyroid goiter with local follicular epithelial dysplasia

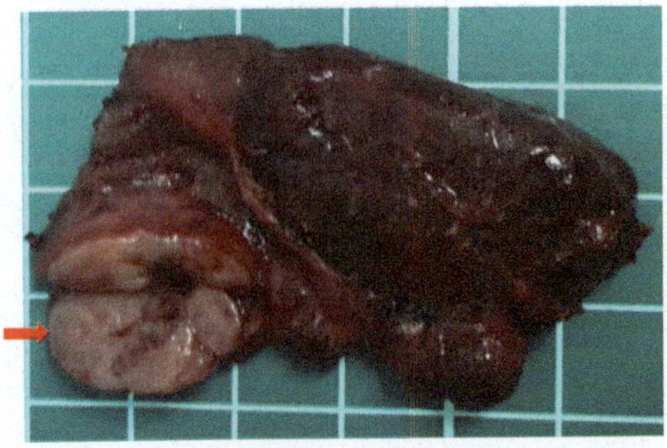

Fig. 1.23 Gross specimen. A 2.0-cm gray-brown nodule could be palpated with a hard texture and a clear margin

ter is prone to occur degenerative changes, with varying degrees of calcification or liquefaction. Usually due to hematoma absorption, mechanization of the nodule wall, or calcification of the fibrous septum after the hemorrhagic cystic degeneration. Ultrasound images show that the calcification foci are usually relatively large, curved, ring-shaped, or plaque-shaped, generally >5 mm in diameter, and the posterior sound and shadow are obvious. Gray-white fibrous cut tape interspersed with nodules or forming the sac wall can often be seen in large specimens of nodular goiter, interspersed with gray-white calcification and ossification (Figs. 1.24, 1.25, 1.26, 1.27, and 1.28).

Case 4

Clinical information: A 44-year-old female patient was detected with a nodule on the left lobe while health examination without clinical symptoms. T3, T4, and TSH levels were normal. Specialized physical examination: A tough nodule about 1.0 cm in the left thyroid lobe could be palpated, which moves up and down along with swallowing.

Ultrasonic information: Sonographic reports in two different institutions: hypoechoic nodule in the left lobe with hyperechoic spots visible inside. First impressions of the clinician, hyperechoic spots were visible inside, whether small or enlarged? Ultrasound suggested confusion, Thus,

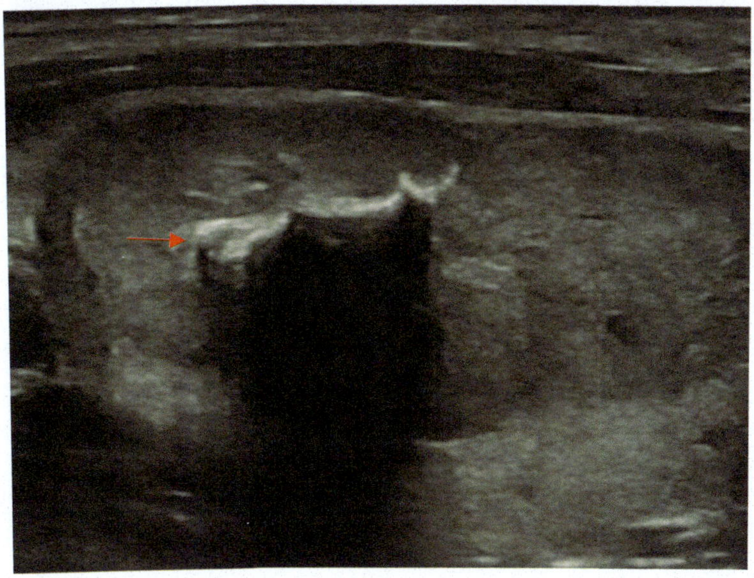

Scan the QR code to watch the ultrasonic video

Fig. 1.24 Hypoechoic mass could be detected in the right lobe with coarse hyperechoic foci inside

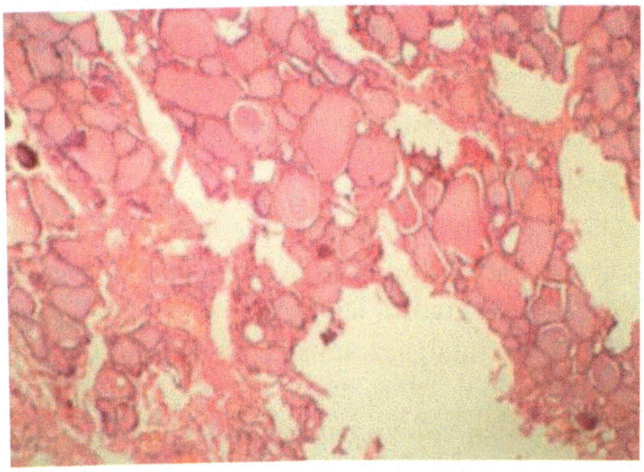

Fig. 1.25 Pathological diagnosis Nodular thyroid goiter shows degenerative changes, with varying degrees of calcification. Pathological diagnosis: nodular goiter with adenoma nodule formation, local vitreous degeneration and calcification

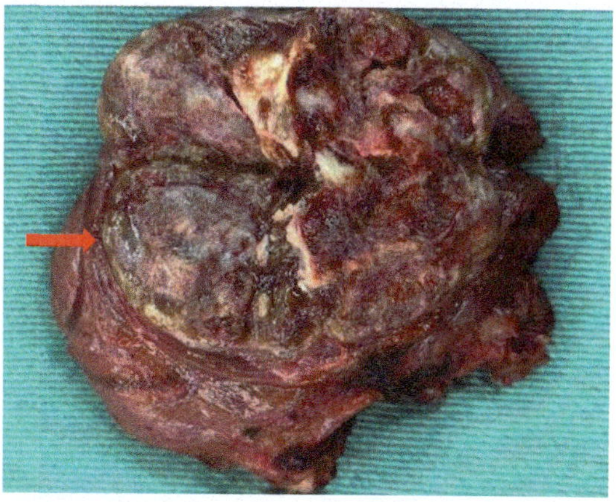

Fig. 1.26 Gross specimen. A 4.0-cm gray-white-gray-yellow nodule with clear margin and focal calcification inside. The incision feeling is hard

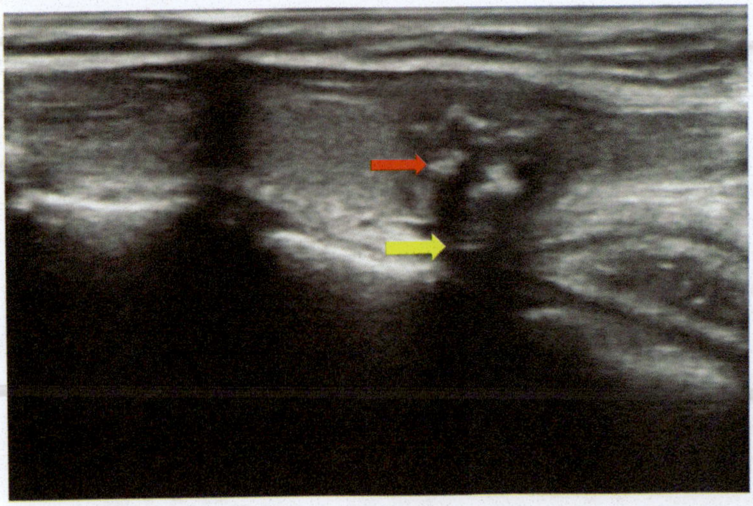

Scan the QR code to watch the ultrasonic video

Fig. 1.27 Hypoechoic mass could be detected in the right lobe with coarse hyperechoic foci inside. Sonograms of nodular goiter show that the calcification foci are usually coarse, curved, ring-shaped, or plaque-shaped, generally >5 mm in diameter, and the posterior acoustic shadowing is bright (yellow arrow). Several large, irregularly shaped hyperechoic foci with a diameter of >2 mm are visible in hypoechoic nodules

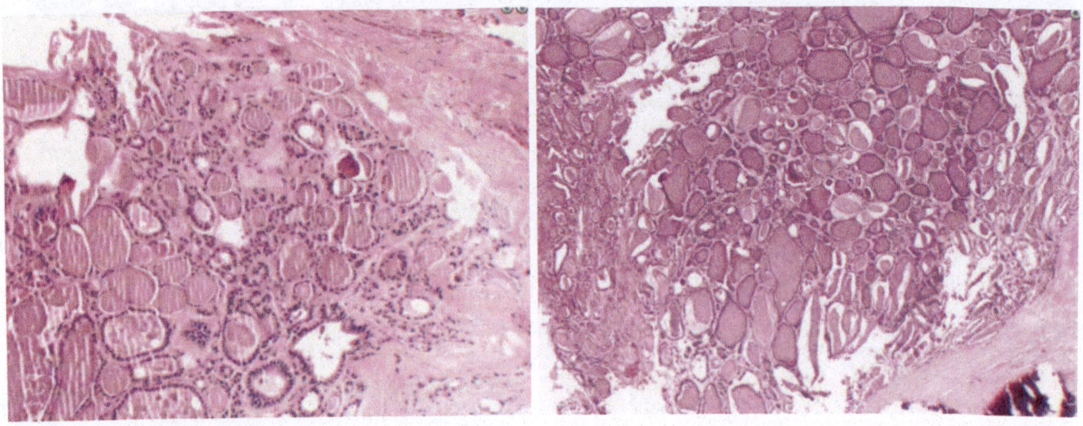

Fig. 1.28 Pathological diagnosis: Nodular thyroid goiter

fine needle aspiration cytology was recommended for this patient (Figs. 1.29 and 1.30).

Preoperative ultrasound evaluation: Fig. 1.31

Gross specimen and pathological diagnosis: Figs. 1.32 and 1.33

Discussion: Misdiagnosis analysis and prevention strategies

The calcification of thyroid nodules is histologically divided into sand granules and malnourished calcifications. Sand granules present microcalcification on ultrasound, which is closely related to papillary thyroid carcinoma. However, the sonographic findings of malnourished calcification are variable. The shape of calcification is mostly irregular, accompanied by posterior echogenicity attenuation, which obscures the internal and posterior structures of calcification, resulting in loss of diagnostic information.

Cyclic calcification is a type of malnourished calcification, distributed around thyroid nodules, and is a special form of calcification. In the past, ring calcification was considered to be related to

Sonographic findings

Right lobe: 5.4 cm × 1.5 cm × 1.2 cm.

Left lobe: 5.0 cm × 1.4 cm × 1.1 cm.

Isthmus: anteroposterior diameter is 0.2 cm.

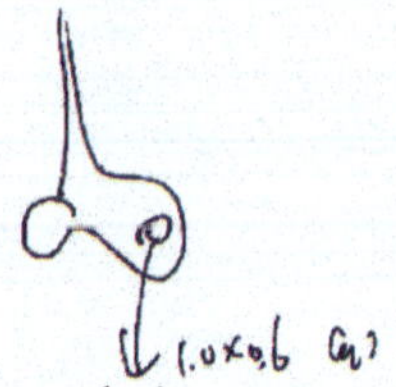

The echogenicity of parenchyma are uniform. A 1.0 cm × 0.6 cm hypoechoic regular margin nodule was detected in the inferior of the left lobe, with regular shape and hyperechogenic foci inside.

CDFI: A small blood flow signal was detected in the aforementioned hypoechoic nodule.

Sonographic indicates:

Hypoechoic areas on the left thyroid lobe with calcification (TI-RADS 3)

Fig. 1.29 Sonographic report of Case 4.1

Sonographic findings

Right lobe: 4.8 cm × 1.6 cm × 1.3 cm.

Left lobe: 4.8 cm × 1.4 cm × 1.0 cm.

Isthmus: anteroposterior diameter is 0.18 cm.

The shape and size were normal on the transverse view, the echogenicity of parenchyma are uniform. A 1.2 cm × 0.5 cm hypoechoic regular margin nodule was detected in the inferior of the left lobe, with regular shape and hyperechogenic foci inside.

CDFI: No blood flow signal was detected in the aforementioned hypoechoic nodule.

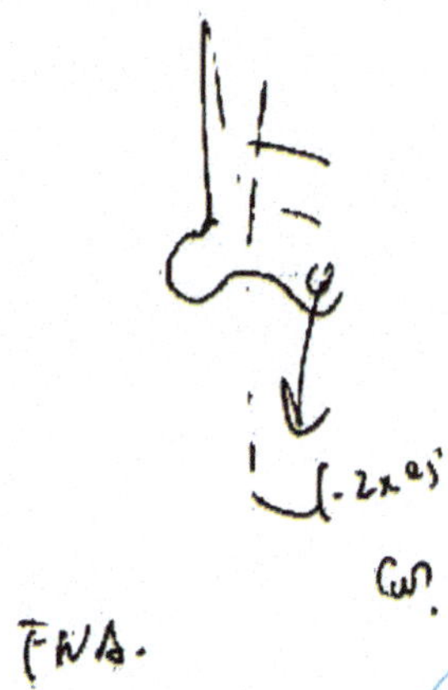

Sonographic indicates:

Hypoechoic areas on the left thyroid lobe with calcification (TI-RADS 3)

Fig. 1.30 Sonographic report of Case 4.2

benign thyroid nodules. With the development of clinical diagnostic techniques (especially high-frequency ultrasound), it was found that the proportion of ring calcifications in malignant nodules has gradually increased.

Coarse and peripheral calcifications are often considered to be a more common sign of benign thyroid lesions. However, both are also present in malignant thyroid nodules, and the mechanism is unknown. Part of the study suggests that it is due to the formation of calcification around the nodes or fibrous strip calcifications after the absorption of inflammatory hematomas.

On the ultrasound sonogram, it is shown as patchy, bar, or surrounding arc calcification in the nodule, often accompanied by echogenicity behind. Some studies have also suggested that it is related to the elevation of local alkaline phos-

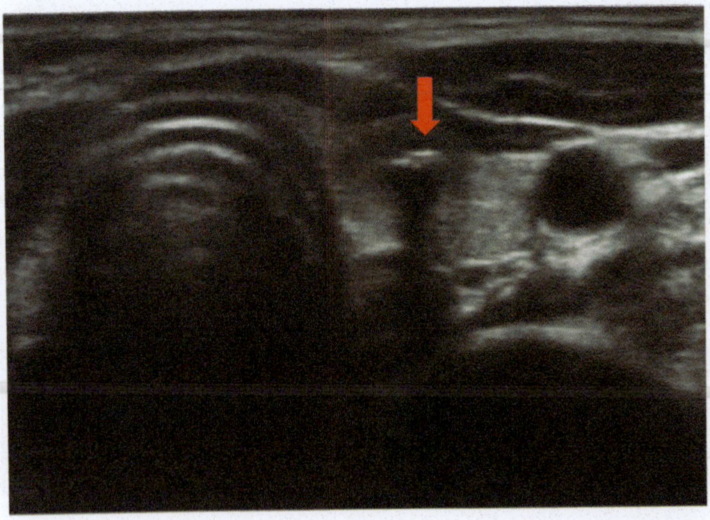

Scan the QR code to watch the ultrasonic video

Fig. 1.31 Preoperative ultrasonic reevaluation. Two linear hyperechoic foci are visible in hypoechoic nodules with acoustic shadowing behind

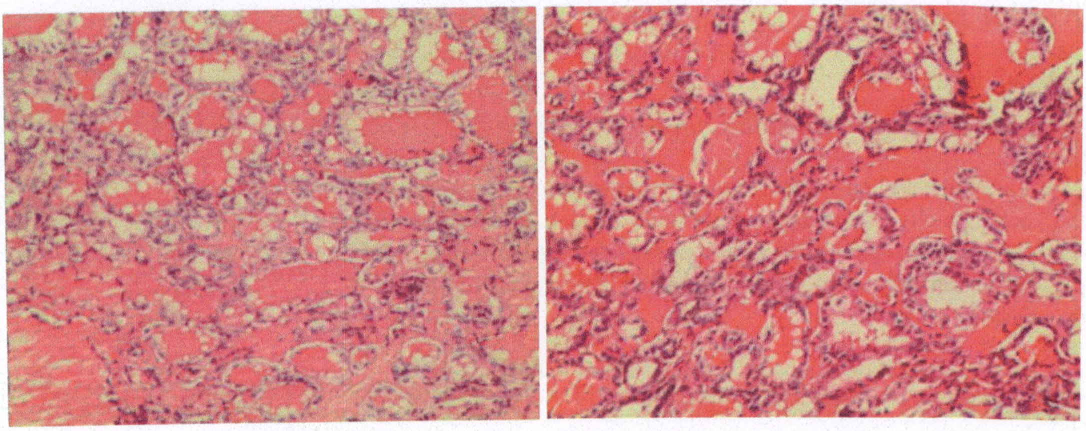

Fig. 1.32 Pathological diagnosis of Case 4. No sand granules are clearly seen under the microscope, so ultrasound shows that short-line hyperechogenicity may be fibrotic hyperplasia. Diagnosis: (left lobe) thyroid papillary microcarcinoma (tumor diameter: 0.8 cm), invading the thyroid capsule. Immunohistochemical examination: CD56(−), CK19 (+), Galectin-3 (+), HBME-1 (+), TPO (−)

phatase, which can hydrolyze organic phosphate esters, resulting in local phosphoric acid exceeding the normal value of 3Ca2+: 2PO43- forming calcium phosphate deposition and leading to calcification. The theories about the formation mechanism are under investigation.

Coarse calcification requires a combination of other ultrasound signs, and it is difficult to judge the benign or malicious nature of the nodule based on calcification alone (Figs. 1.34, 1.35, and 1.36).

Case 5

Clinical information: A 14-year-old male patient presented with left cervical mass accidentally with uncomfortable swallowing. T3, T4, and TSH levels were present in Table 1.2. Specialized physical examination: A tough nodule about 2.0 cm in the left thyroid lobe could be palpated, which moves up and down along with swallowing. Nothing could be palpated in the right lobe.

Ultrasonic information: Hyperechoic mass can be detected in the left thyroid lobe. Owing to the young age and the hyperechoic nodule, fine needle aspiration cytology was recommended for this patient (Fig. 1.37).

Preoperative ultrasound evaluation: Fig. 1.38

Gross specimen and pathological diagnosis: Figs. 1.39, 1.40 and 1.41

Discussion: Misdiagnosis analysis and prevention strategies

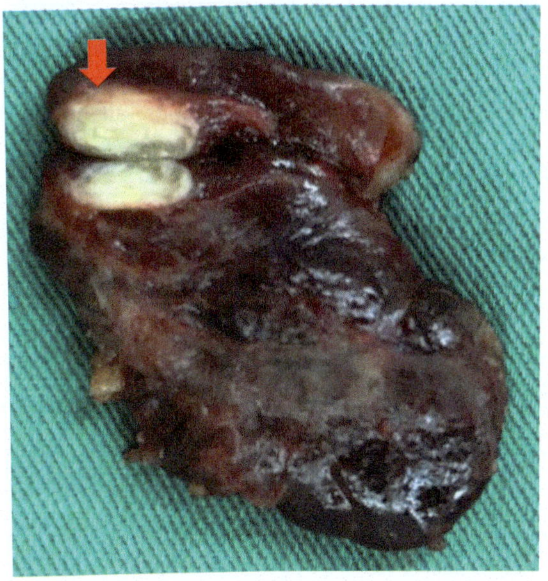

Fig. 1.33 Gross specimen of case 4. A 0.8-cm hard nodule could be palpated on the thyroid capsule with gray-white in cross-section and clear margin (red arrow)

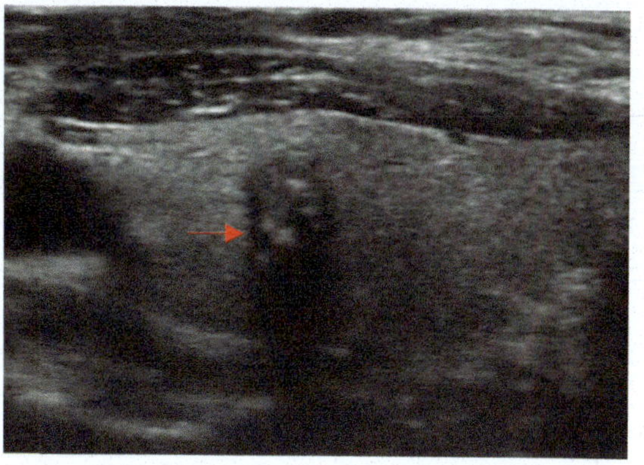

Fig. 1.34 Hyperechoic foci could be detected with a diameter >2 mm. Combined with other signs of ultrasound (hypoechogenicity, taller than wide), the risk of malignancy for the nodule increased. Pathological diagnosis: thyroid papillary microcarcinoma

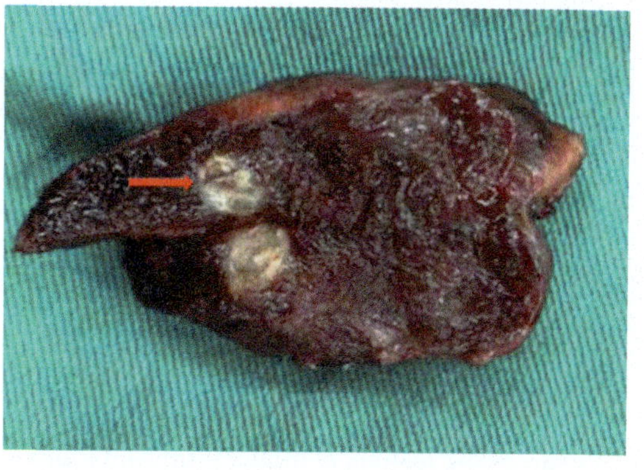

Fig. 1.35 Gross specimen

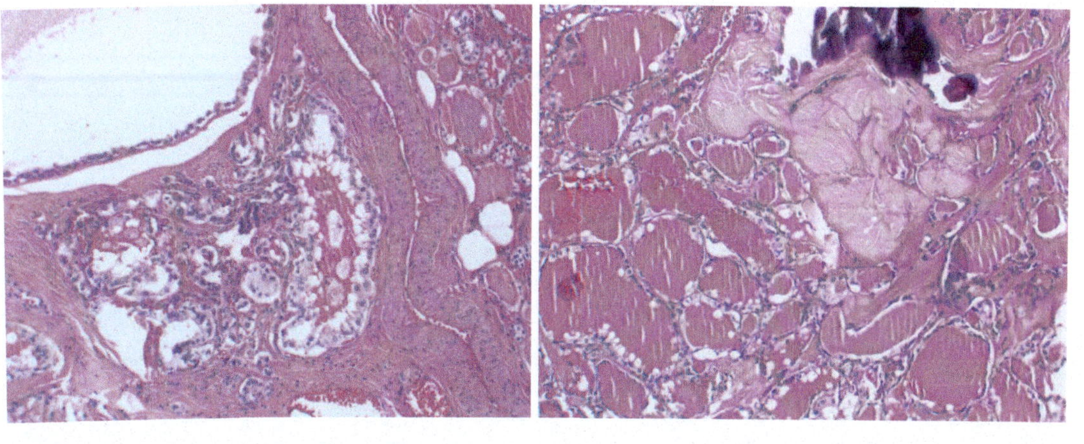

Fig. 1.36 Pathological diagnosis. Size of tumor: 0.7 cm, 0.1 cm; histological type: thyroid papillary microcarcinoma

Diffuse sclerosing variant of papillary thyroid carcinoma (DSVPTC) is a rare, special type of papillary thyroid carcinoma that is common in young patients and presents as thyroid goiter without a characteristic mass. Diffuse fibrous tissue hyperplasia, sclerosis, focal or diffuse lymphatic cell infiltration, a large number of sand granules, atypical papilla formation, and squamous epithelial metaplasia are the main pathological features, accounting for 0.7%–6.6% of papillary thyroid carcinoma.

Table 1.2 Hormone level of thyroid function

Hormone	Value	Normal value	Unit
FT3	3.36	3.21–6.5	pmol/L
FT_4	7.68	10.20–21.88	pmol/L
TSH	>100.0	10.20–21.88	μU/mL
ATG	>5000	0–72	U/mL
A-TPO	>2000	0–72	U/mL

Clinical characteristics: DSVPTC tends to harbor extrathyroidal extension, and often metastasizes to lymph nodes and lungs, and can also be transferred to the brain, bone. DSVPTC is aggressive and metastasize early concomitant with poor prognosis. The incidence of the DSVPTC is low, the clinical manifestations are insidious, and thyroid

Sonographic findings:

Right lobe: 4.8 cm × 1.6 cm × 1.3 cm. Left lobe: 4.8 cm × 1.4 cm × 1.0 cm. Isthmus: anteroposterior diameter is 0.18 cm. The thickened and enhanced light spot in thyroid parenchyma are uniform. Two anechoic dark areas were seen in the right lobe, one of which was 0.2 cm × 0.2 cm. A 2.4 cm × 1.3 cm hyperechoic ill-defined margin nodule was detected in the left lobe, with mild protrusion effect on transverse view. And a 0.7 cm × 0.6 cm hypoechoic mass was detected.

CDFI: Linear blood flow signals could be seen in the left nodule and surroundings.

Sonographic indicates:

Uniform thyroid parenchyma

Solid mass in the left lobe, suggest further examination

Small cystic lesions in bilateral thyroid lobes

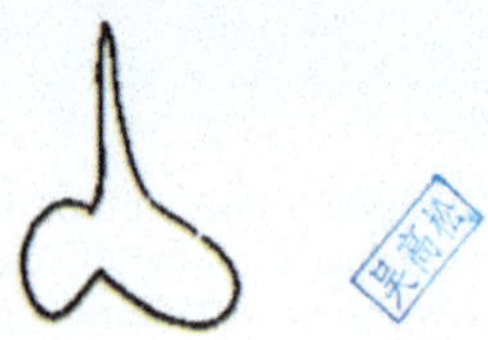

Fig. 1.37 Sonographic report of Case 5

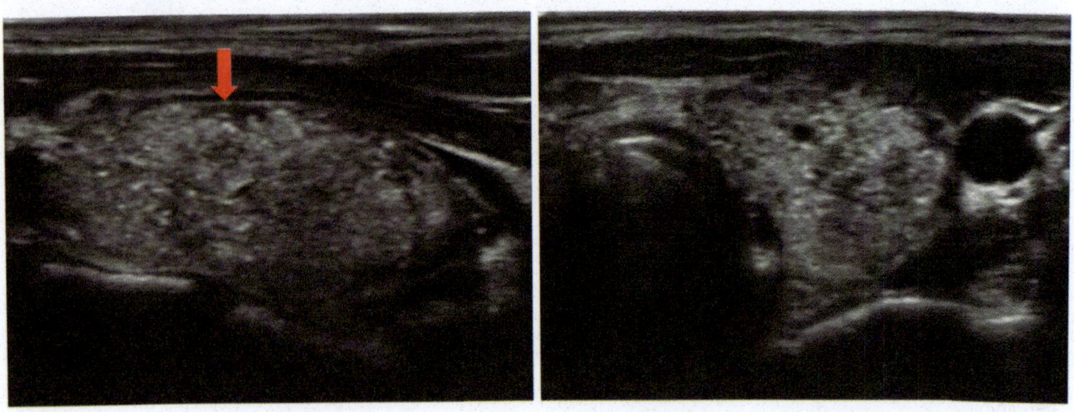

Fig. 1.38 Preoperative ultrasonic reevaluation of Case 5. Diffuse enlargement of the left lobe and diffuse punctate hyperechogenicity ("blizzards") could be observed interspersed with hypoechoic areas

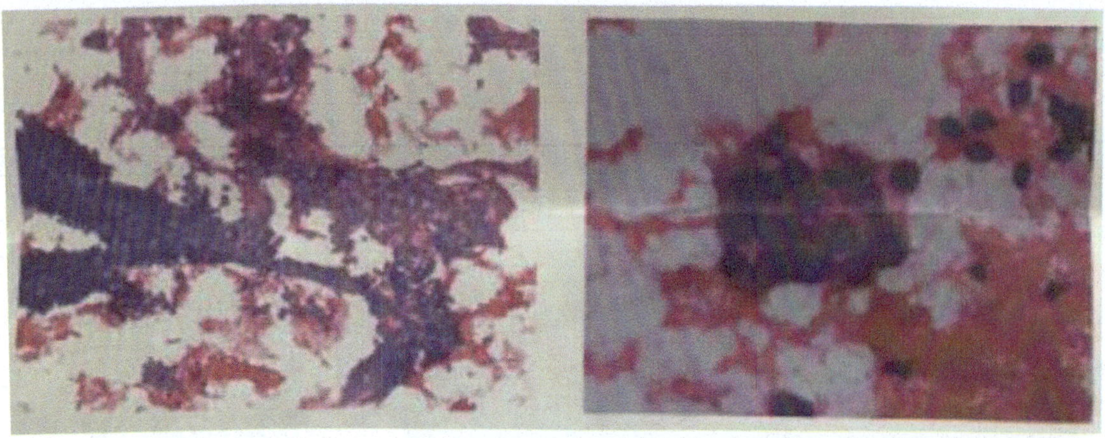

Fig. 1.39 Reports of fine needle aspiration cytology for Case 5: papillary thyroid carcinoma

Fig. 1.40 Gross specimen of Case 5. The left lobe is palpated hard. Resect the gland along the hardest area. A 2-cm lesion was observed with an ill-defined margin

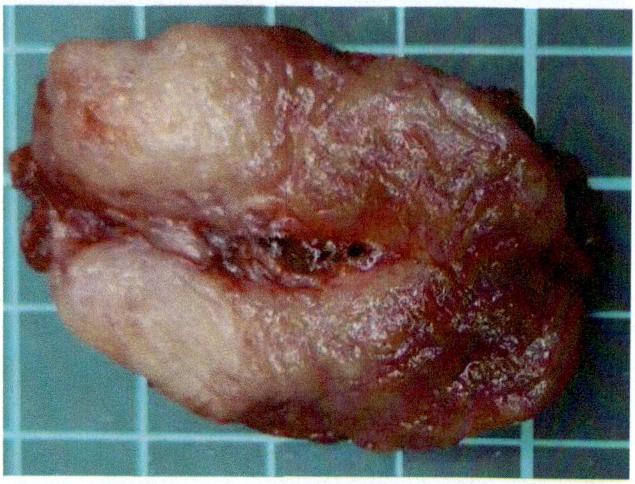

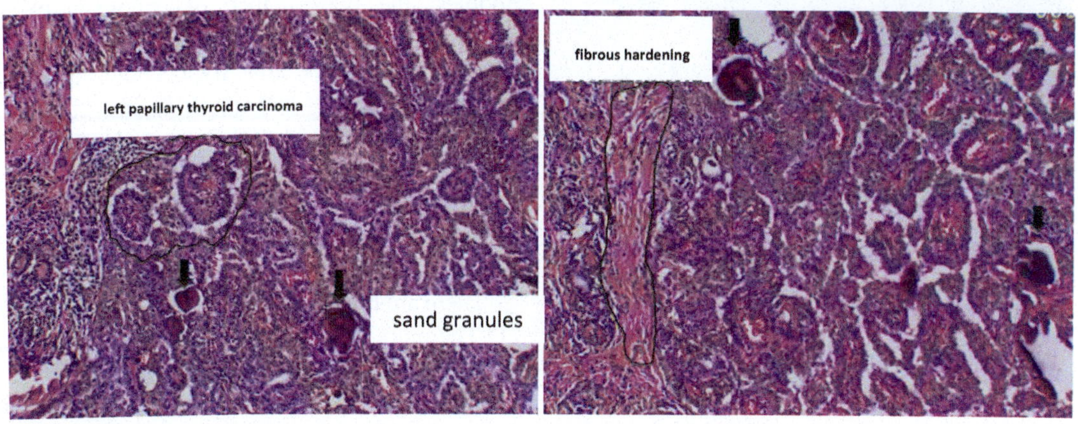

Fig. 1.41 Pathological diagnosis of Case 5. Microscopic sand granules (black arrows), fibrous hyperplasia, hardening, atypical papillary formation. Pathological diagnosis: left papillary thyroid carcinoma (maximum diameter 2.0 cm). Tumor invaded dorsal membrane, no obvious intraveal carcinoma embolism and nerve invasion was observed

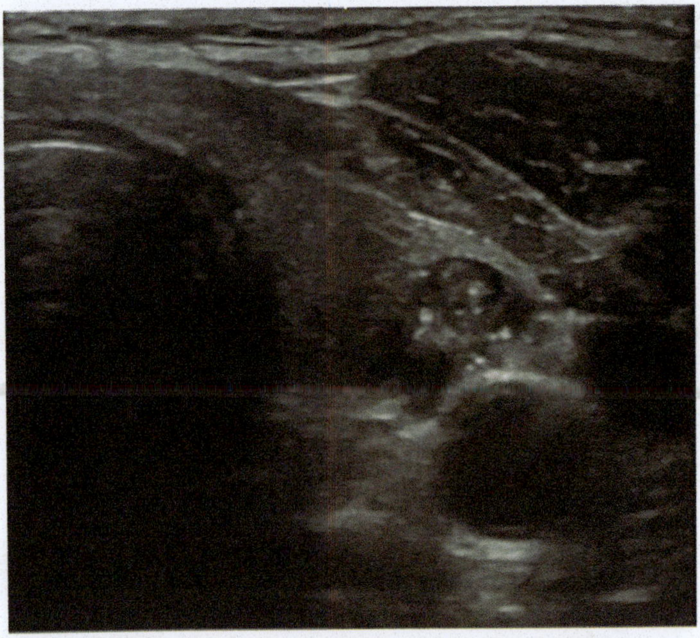

Scan the QR code
to watch the ultrasonic video

Fig. 1.42 A 45-year-old male patient with a 1.4 cm × 1.0 cm hypoechoic nodule with hyperechoic foci in the left lobe. Diagnosis: nodular thyroid goiter with adenoma nodule formation (concentrated colloid present punctate hyperechogenicity with a comet-tail sign behind)

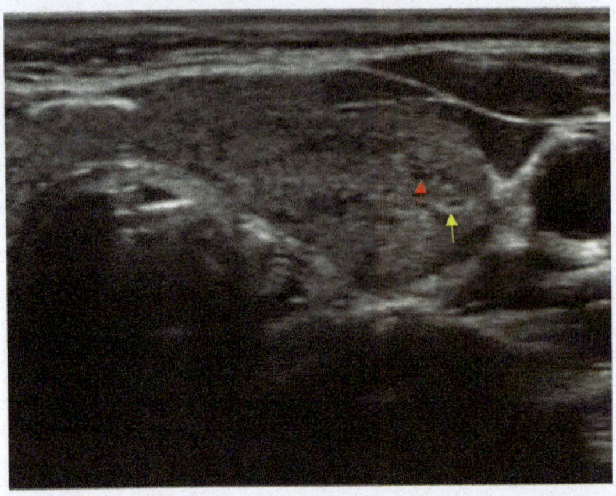

Fig. 1.43 A 46-year-old female patient with uneven parenchyma in the left thyroid lobe, interspersed with hypoechoic nodules of varying sizes, and hyperechogenicity foci were observed. Diagnosis: Hashimoto's thyroiditis

nodules are difficult to be palpated. Mild or moderate enlargement of unilateral or bilateral lobes of the tough thyroid gland with a rough surface and unobvious tenderness are the clinical manifestation. Enlarged hard lymph nodes can be palpated in the anterior and lateral cervical areas. Ultrasound physicians and surgeons are prone to misdiagnosis due to their lack of experience with this disease.

The main manifestations of DSVPTC ultrasound are: (1) diffuse microcalcification, showing "blizzard" signs; (2) uneven areas similar to nodules, the performance of echogenicity is diverse, without a clear mass effect; (3) tumor nodules tend to be low hypoechoic; and (4) hyperechoic lesions can appear in part of gland. Patients with diffuse sclerosing papillary thyroid carcinoma have a diffuse distribution of microcalcifications in clusters of accumulation in the thyroid parenchyma, which is the only indication and contains great diagnostic significance.

There are four causes of misdiagnosis of DSV: (1) There are no obvious nodules and masses in the enlarged thyroid gland. (2) DSV coexists with benign nodules, which obscures the diagnosis of DSV. (3) The characteristics of sandy granular calcification in the thyroid gland are not significant and should be distinguished from Hashimoto's thyroiditis, concentrated colloidal substances, small calcifications on the blood vessel wall, and dense fibrosis. (4) The pathological characteristics of DSVPTC are diffuse involvement of one or two lobes of the thyroid gland. Owing to the contamination with Hashimoto's thyroiditis. DSVPTC tends to be misdiagnosed as Hashimoto's thyroiditis. Hashimoto's thyroid glands have diffuse hypoechogenicity with scattered strip hyperechogenicity without clusters or diffuse microcalcifications in the affected gland. Concentrated colloid substances show punctate hyperechogenicity with Comet-tail sign behind that can be distinguished from microcalcifications (Figs. 1.42 and 1.43). Therefore, it is particularly important to improve the awareness of clinicians and ultrasound physicians about this disease. The echogenicity thyroid parenchymal is messy and cannot be simply diagnosed as inflammatory changes, and DSVPTC is a rare type of high degree of malignancy that should be highly suspected to avoid patients missing the best opportunity for surgery.

Further Readings

Haugen BR, Alexander EK, Bible KC, Doherty GM, Mandel SJ, Nikiforov YE, Pacini F, Randolph GW, Sawka AM, Schlumberger M, Schuff KG, Sherman SI, Sosa JA, Steward DL, Tuttle RM, Wartofsky L. American Thyroid Association management guidelines for adult patients with thyroid nodules and differentiated thyroid cancer: the American Thyroid Association Guidelines Task Force on thyroid nodules and differentiated thyroid cancer. Thyroid. 2016;26(1):1–133.

Lu Z, Mu Y, Zhu H, et al. Clinical value of using ultrasound to assess calcification patterns in thyroid nodules. World J Surg. 2011;35(1):122–7.

Tessler FN, Middleton WD, Grant EG, Hoang JK, Berland LL, Teefey SA, Cronan JJ, Beland MD, Desser TS, Frates MC, Hammers LW, Hamper UM, Langer JE, Reading CC, Scoutt LM, Stavros AT. ACR thyroid imaging, reporting and data system (TI-RADS): white paper of the ACR TI-RADS Committee. J Am Coll Radiol. 2017;14(5):587–95.

2 Crystals in Glial Thyroid Cyst

The thyroid is the largest endocrine gland in the human body and contains many round or oval acinar vesicles of varying sizes. The acinar vesicle is surrounded by monolayer epithelial cells, and the acinar cavity is filled with colloid. Colloid are the secretion of acinar epithelial cells, the main component of which is thyroglobulin. After the hyperplasia of thyroid follicle, a large number of colloids would be produced, and the colloid would be highly concentrated in the nodules, which is manifested on ultrasound as punctate hyperechogenicity in cystic nodule with comet-tail sign behind (Fig. 2.1), which is a kind of artifact on ultrasound image and is the result of multiple mixing sounds. Colloidal nodules may contain tiny crystals produced by dried colloids, the acoustic reflection of the crystals produces a bright point, the suspended crystals begin to vibrate under the influence of ultrasonic energy, the vibrations produce sound waves, and the sound waves return to the ultrasound probe after the initial reflection signal. Comet-tail sign helps to distinguish typical benign calcifications found in colloidal nodules from highly suspected microcalcifications. When a single comet-tail sign appears in a small colloid cyst, similar to the human eye, which is called "eyeball sign" (Fig. 2.2).

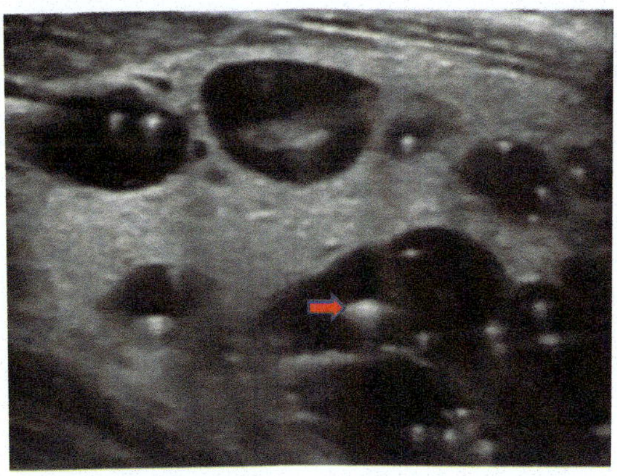

Fig. 2.1 Comet-tail sign

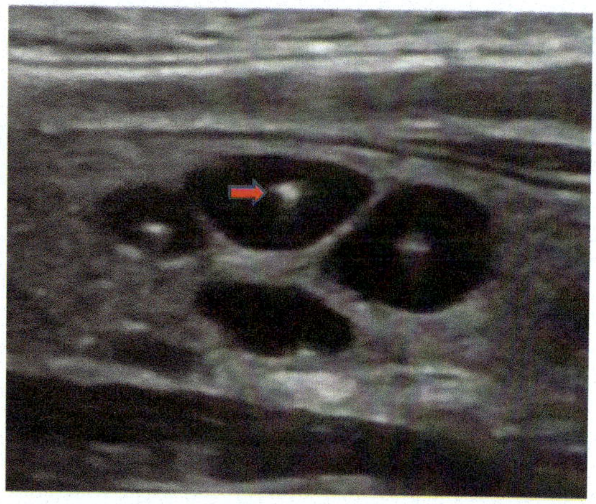

Fig. 2.2 Eyeball sign. When a separate comet-tail sign appears in a small colloidal cyst, the manifestation is similar to the human eye, called the "eyeball sign"

G. Wu et al., *Pitfalls in Ultrasound of Thyroid Nodules*,
https://doi.org/10.1007/978-981-19-8873-8_2

Case 6

Ultrasonic information: Fig. 2.3

Ultrasonic information: Fig. 2.4

Case 7

Clinical information: A 60-year-old male patient presented with cervical mass for two years. T3, T4, and TSH levels were normal. Specialized physical examination: A tough nodule about 1.0 cm × 0.7 cm in the left thyroid lobe could be palpated, which moves up and down along with swallowing.

Ultrasonic information: Fig. 2.5

Preoperative ultrasound evaluation: Fig. 2.6

Gross specimen and pathological diagnosis: Figs. 2.7 and 2.8

Discussion: Misdiagnosis analysis and prevention strategies

Thyroid ultrasonography reveals hyperechoic lesions in 23% of nodules, which may be microcalcifications with high specificity for diagnosing malignancy or maybe the concentrated colloid with comet-tail sign. The concentrated colloid in benign thyroid tumors form tiny crystals that can

Ultrasonic images:

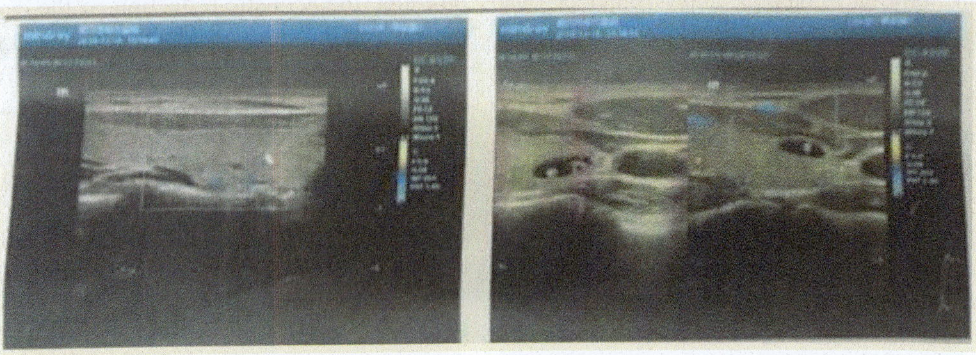

Sonographic findings:

Size and shape were normal for the bilateral thyroid lobes. Right lobe: 3.9 cm × 1.3 cm × 1.0 cm. Left lobe: 3.9 cm × 1.1 cm × 1.0 cm. Isthmus: anteroposterior diameter is 0.25 cm. Thyroid envelope is smooth and the echogenicity of parenchyma are uniform.

Several hypoechoic areas were seen in the left lobe, one of which was 0.96 cm × 0.39 cm with clear margin and punctate hyperechogenicity inside. A 0.13 cm × 0.10 cm cystic anechoic area with clear margin.

CDFI: No blood flow signals could be detected.

Sonographic indicates:

Hypoechoic nodule in the left lobe with calcification, suggest regular follow-up

Fig. 2.3 Sonographic report of Case 6.1. A 30-year-old female patient presented with eyeball sign, which was tend to be benign nodule, and regular follow-up was recommended. A 30-year-old female patient presented with eyeball sign, which was tend to be benign nodule, and regular follow-up was recommended

Ultrasonic images:

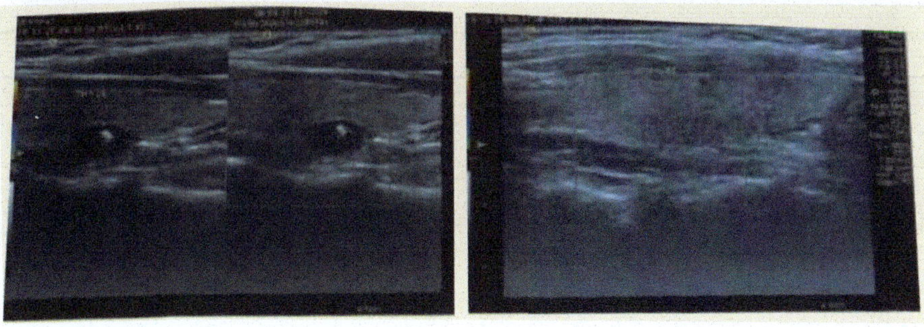

Sonographic findings:

Thyroid scan:

Right lobe: 5.7 cm × 1.6 cm × 1.3 cm.

Left lobe: 5.3 cm × 1.6 cm × 1.4 cm.

Isthmus: anteroposterior diameter is 0.14 cm.

Size and shape were normal on thyroid transverse view. The echogenicity of parenchyma is uneven. An anechoic 0.9 cm × 0.6 cm area with clear margin and hyperechoic spots inside in the middle dorsal of left lobe. No obvious limited echogenicity was detected in the right lobe.

CDFI: No blood flow signals could be detected.

Sonographic indicates:

Anechoic area in the left lobe (colloid cyst ?)

Fig. 2.4 Sonographic report of Case 6.2. A 33-year-old female patient presented with eyeball sign, which was tend to be benign nodule, and regular follow-up was recommended

be manifested as punctate hyperechogenicity on ultrasound. Microcalcification refers to circular stratified calcium deposit crystals with a diameter of 10–100 μm, equivalent to gravel histopathologically, and can present punctate hyperechogenicity in ultrasound. Influenced by low resolution of instrument, diagnostician cognition and judgment ability and many other factors, many punctate hyperechogenicity in nodules are misdiagnosed as microcalcification.

Comet-tail sign is a manifestation of multiple reflection artifacts, the form is mostly inverted triangle, the display rate of which is related to the device adjustment. The adjustment of instrument may increase or decrease the comet-tail sign during operation. The formation of comet-tail sign is closely related to a large number of colloids, which usually appear in benign nodules, so comet-tail sign may be benign sign. However, not all the punctate hyperechogenicity with comet-

Ultrasonic images:

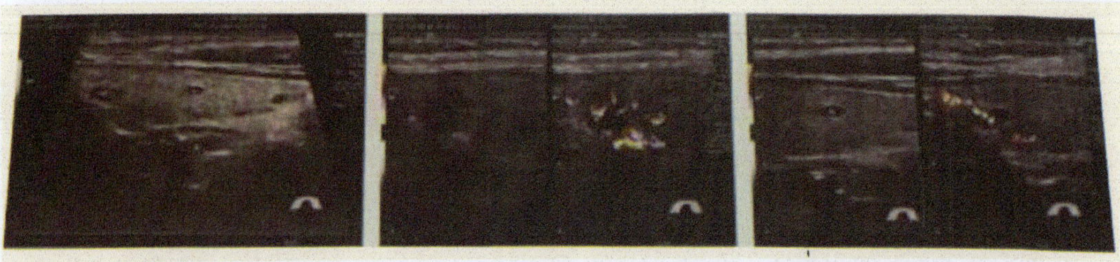

Sonographic findings:

Thyroid scan:

Right lobe: 4.3 cm × 1.2 cm × 1.1 cm.

Left lobe: 3.4 cm × 1.5 cm × 1.1 cm.

Isthmus: anteroposterior diameter is 0.35 cm.

Size and shape were normal on thyroid transverse view. The echogenicity of parenchyma are uneven.

Several hypoechoic ill-defined margin areas were seen in the right lobe with uneven echogenicity and hyperechoic spots inside, one of which was 0.8 cm × 0.5 cm with blood flow signal.

A hypoechoic 0.5 cm × 0.3 cm area with clear margin and uneven echogenicity inside, without blood flow signal.

Several anechoic areas could be detected in the bilateral lobes with clear margin and posterior hyperechogenicity, one of which was 0.4 cm × 0.2 cm in size, without blood flow signal.

Sonographic indicates:

Hypoechoic nodule in the right lobe with calcification (TI-RADS 4a).

Hypoechoic nodule in the left lobe (TI-RADS 3).

Cystic masses in bilateral thyroid lobes (TI-RADS 2)

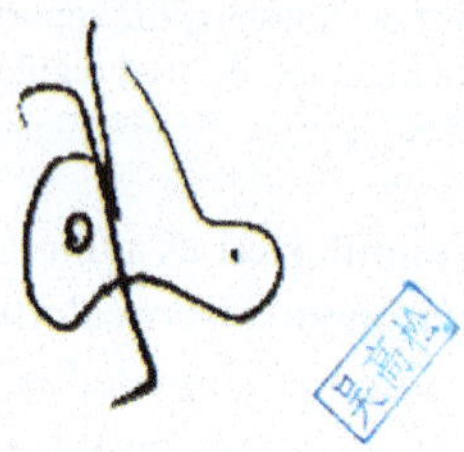

Fig. 2.5 Sonographic report of Case 7

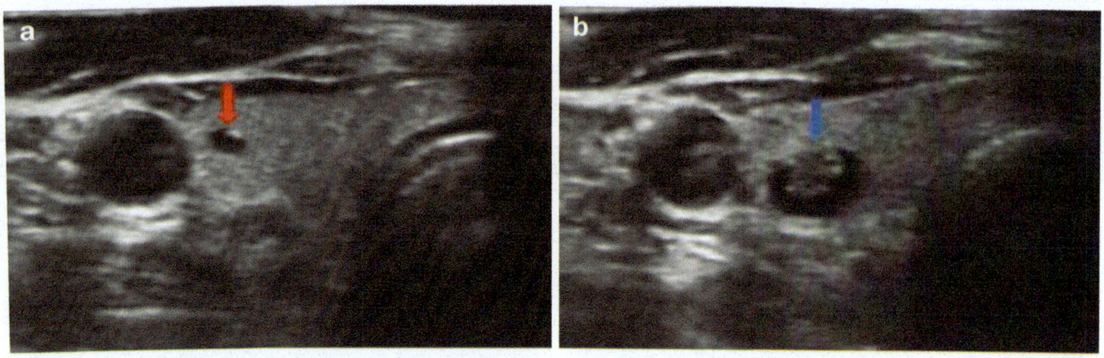

Fig. 2.6 Preoperative ultrasonic reevaluation. (**A**) Hypoechoic foci in the superior right lobe could be detected with punctate hyperechogenicity inside (red arrow, TI-RADS 2); (**B**) A 0.8 cm × 0.5 cm hypoechoic nodule in the inferior right lobe with several hyperechoic foci inside (blue arrow, TI-RADS 4a)

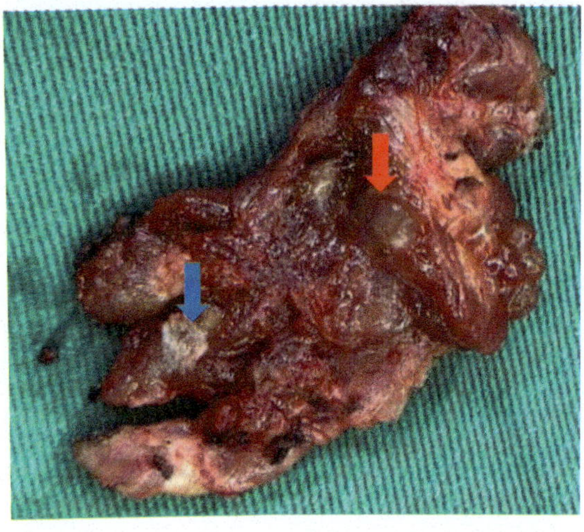

Fig. 2.7 Gross specimen of Case 7. The section of the red arrow nodule specimen is jelly-shaped, and the pathological diagnosis is nodule thyroid goiter. The blue arrow nodule specimen is grayish white, qualitative hard, and the pathological diagnosis is thyroid papillary microcarcinoma

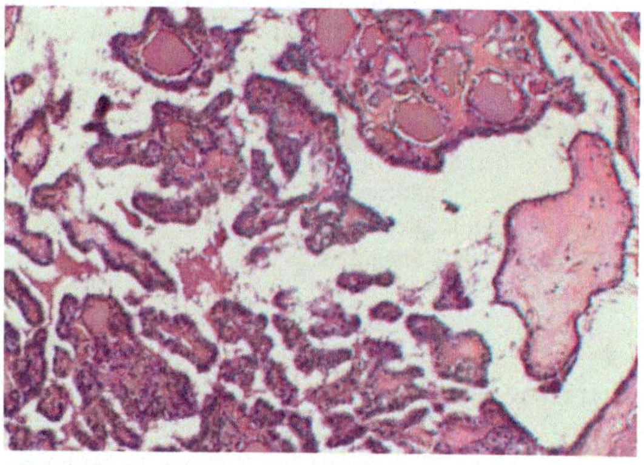

Fig. 2.8 Pathological diagnosis Case 7. Pathological diagnosis: thyroid papillary microcarcinoma

tail signs is concentrated colloid. Similarly, the punctate hyperechogenicity caused by concentrated colloid may not be accompanied by a comet-tail sign.

Ahuja et al. found that only 80% of nodules with comet-tail signs are filled with colloids, and the remaining hyperechogenicity foci produce comet-tail signs may be related to necrotic debris after adenoma bleeding, and this study infers that the comet-tail signs in cystic nodules are benign signs (Fig. 2.9). Malhi et al. believe that all types of hyperechogenicity foci, except those with large comet-tail sign artifacts, are related to malignant tumors. Wu et al. consider that there may also be colloid inside the nodules of papillary thyroid carcinoma, and that the ultrasonic sonogram will show the microcyst structure in the part of the nodule, the punctate hyperechogenicity (Fig. 2.10) and the comet-tail sign behind, which may be the posterior increase strong effect of the posterior wall of the microcapsular, or the ringing artifacts caused by the precipitates that are flattened on the posterior wall of the microcapsular. This manifestation results from microvesicles formed by concentrated colloid, which can be detected in both benign and malignant tumors.

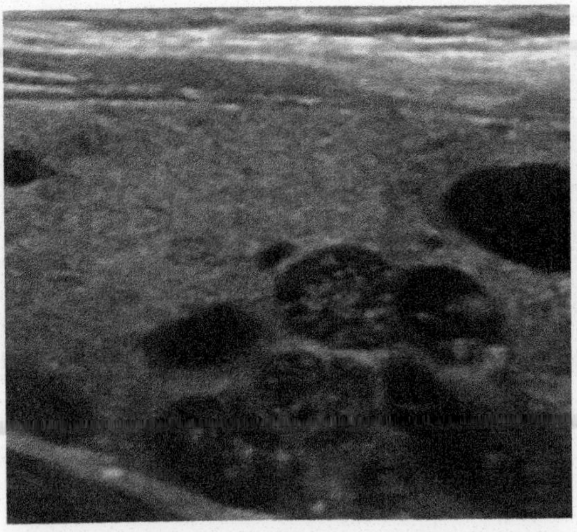

Fig. 2.9 Multiple comet caudal signs and strong dotted echoes can be seen within the nodules, among which dot strong echoes without comet-tail signs may be mistaken for microcalcium. Attention should be paid to the background of the nodules in which they are located, whether they are microcystic areas or solid nodules. Only the comet-tail sign located in the liquefied or junction region can be considered a benign sign

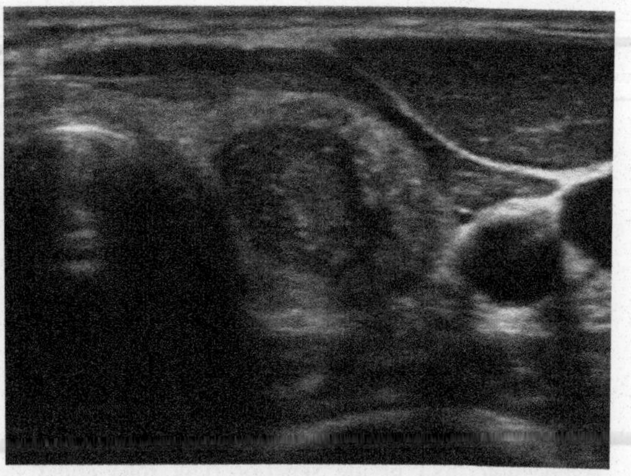

Fig. 2.10 Microcalcification of papillary thyroid carcinoma. Compared with the Fig. 2.9, the punctate strong echo foci shown by microcalcification are usually seen in solid nodules, while comet-tail signs are common in cystic or microcystic areas

Further Readings

Ahuja A, Chick W, King W, et al. Clinical significance of the comet-tail artifact in thyroid ultrasound. J Clin Ultrasound. 1996;24(3):129–33.

Hongxun W, Bingjie Z, Jie L, et al. Echogenic foci with comet-tail artifact in resected thyroid nodules: not an absolute predictor of benign disease. PLoS One. 2018;13(1):e0191505.

Malhi H, Beland MD, Cen SY, et al. Echogenic foci in thyroid nodules: significance of posterior acoustic artifacts. Am J Roentgenol. 2014;203(6):1310–6.

Tahvildari AM, Pan M, Kong CS, et al. Sonographic pathologic correlation for punctate echogenic reflectors in papillary thyroid carcinoma. What are they? J Ultrasound Med. 2016;35(8):1645–52.

3 Mummified Thyroid Nodules

Nodular thyroid goiter is the most common benign thyroid tumor, formed by the repeated stimulation of thyroid-stimulating hormone to thyroid gland for a long time, causing fibrous tissue between the follicles hyperplasia, space wrapping, and the formation of nodular lesions of different sizes. If the nodule is too large to compress the surrounding venous, resulting in local blood circulation disorders, tissue ischemia, secondary degeneration, and due to insufficient blood supply, occurring second necrosis, interstitial congestion edema, and cystic changes. If a blood vessel is ruptured, it is combined with bleeding. The contents of the capsule include thick colloidal gelatinous, bloody brown liquid, or chocolate-colored liquid. Ultrasound shows punctate hyperechogenicity in the capsule with a comet-tail sign. The cystic components of the nodule are gradually absorbed over time, resulting in atrophy of the lesion, internal fibrosis, and microcalcification, forming "zombie" nodules, which are characterized by some malignant nodules on the ultrasound, similar to papillary thyroid carcinoma.

Supplementary Information The online version contains supplementary material available at https://doi.org/10.1007/978-981-19-8873-8_3.

G. Wu et al., *Pitfalls in Ultrasound of Thyroid Nodules*,
https://doi.org/10.1007/978-981-19-8873-8_3

Case 8

Ultrasonic information: Figs. 3.1, 3.2, and 3.3

Ultrasonic images:

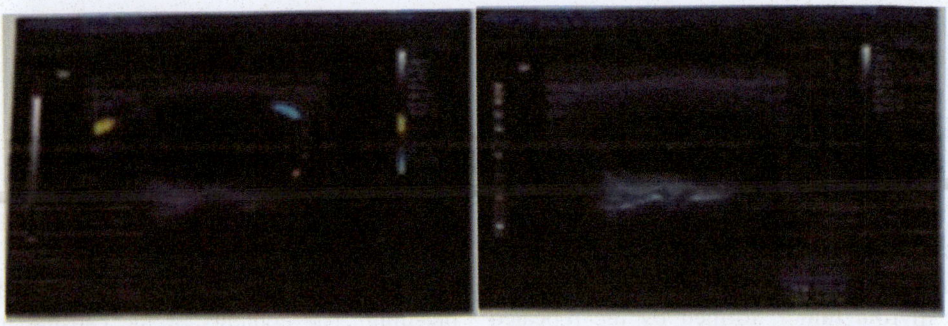

Sonographic findings:

Thyroid scan

Size and shape were normal on thyroid transverse view. The echogenicity of parenchyma are uneven. A 2.6 cm × 1.6 cm × 1.8 cm mixed echoic mass could be detected in the left lobe with regular shape, clear margin and mainly anechoic area inside. No abnormal echogenicity was detected in the right lobe and isthmus.

CDFI: Blood flow signal could be detected around the aforementioned mixed echoic mass.

Sonographic indicates:

A cystic solid nodule in the left lobe, mainly in cystic. (TI-RADS 3)

Fig. 3.1 Sonographic report of Case 8 (2019-7-19). A 35-year-old female patient detected a cystic mixed echoic 2.6 cm × 1.6 cm nodule in the left lobe. Regular follow-up was recommended

Ultrasonic images:

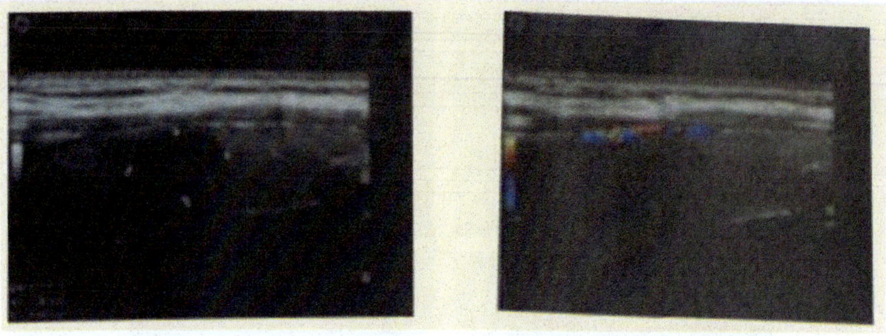

Sonographic findings:

Thyroid scan

Size and shape were normal on thyroid transverse view. The echogenicity of parenchyma is uneven. A 1.4 cm × 0.9 cm hypoechoic area could be detected in the left lobe with clear margin and uneven echogenicity inside. No abnormal echogenicity was detected in the right lobe and isthmus.

No significantly enlarged lymph nodes were detected in central and lateral neck.

CDFI: Blood flow signal could be detected in the hypoechoic area.

Sonographic indicates:

Parenchymal lesion in left lobe (TI-RADS 3)

Fig. 3.2 Sonographic report of Case 8 (2019-10-20). A 1.4 cm × 0.9 cm hypoechoic nodule in the left lobe. Continue regular follow-up was recommended

Ultrasonic images:

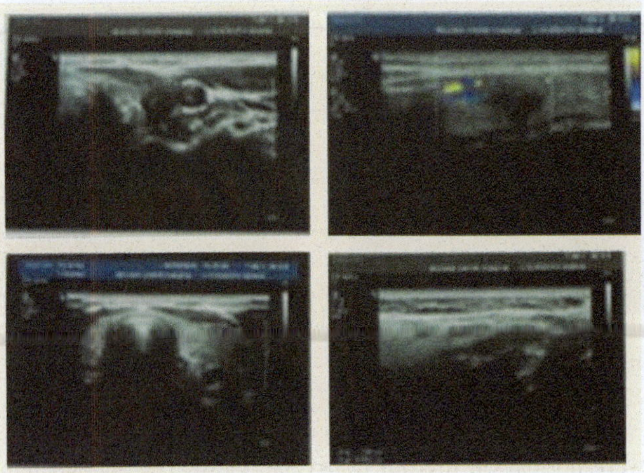

Apply for examination: Thyroid superficial lymph nodes / neck

Sonographic findings:

Size and shape were normal on thyroid transverse view. A 13.2 mm × 8.3 mm × 9.2 mm hypoechoic area could be detected in the upper middle left lobe with ill-defined margin and several hyperechogenicities inside, one of which was 1.7 mm in size.

CDFI: Blood flow signal could be detected around the hypoechoic nodule.

Abnormal echogenicity was detected in bilateral lymph nodes. Lymph nodes in both left and level II were seen, 19.3 mm × 3.8 mm, 19.3 mm × 5.5 mm in size, respectively.

CDFI: Blood flow signal could be detected in the lymph nodes.

Sonographic indicates:

A hypoechoic nodule in left lobe with hyperechoic foci inside (calcification?)

Further examination of bilateral cervical lymph nodes is recommended if necessary

Fig. 3.3 Sonographic report of Case 8 (2020-04-22). Compared with the previous two sonographic reports, size of the nodule did not change, sonographic findings of this taller than wide nodule showed malignant signs with ill-defined margin and several hyperechoic foci inside. Surgery is recommended in another institution. Through periodic sonographic examination, the changes in this nodule are dynamically observed. The cystic solid nodule tends to show hypoechogenicity and microcalcification after being absorbed and dehydrated, which is easily confused with the sonogram of papillary thyroid carcinoma. Dynamic observation is recommended for this patient

Case 9

Ultrasonic information: Figs. 3.4, 3.5, 3.6, and 3.7

Pathological diagnosis: Fig. 3.8

Discussion: Misdiagnosis analysis and prevention strategies: Zombie nodules, also known as post-absorption cyst phenomena, mostly come from cystic solid nodules and cystic nodules after absorption and dehydration, existing very low hypoechogenicity, coarse calcification, blurred margin, and are easily confused with papillary thyroid carcinoma. Persistent shrinkage of previous cysts, shrinkage absorption tendencies of nodules, absence of blood flow signals detected in nodules, and changes in the superposition of contents can be distinguished. Therefore, for the diagnosis of "zombie" nodules, regular ultrasound examination is very important.

Ultrasonic images:

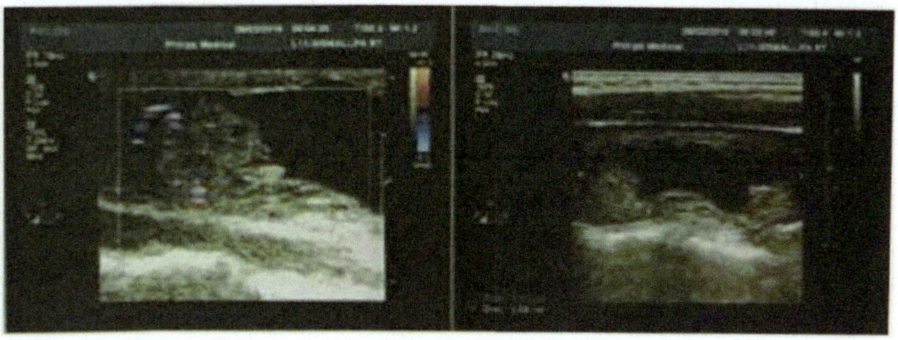

Sonographic findings:

Left lobe: 5.8 cm × 2.6 cm × 1.9 cm;

Right lobe: 5.4 cm × 1.9 cm × 1.7 cm;

Isthmus: anteroposterior diameter is 0.13 cm.

The shape of the thyroid gland was irregular, several liquid anechoic areas were detected inside with uneven wall thicknesses, one of which was 3.6 cm ×1.5 cm ×2.0cm in the left lobe.

Bilateral ultrasound scan: Several lymph nodes were detected, one of which was 2.6 cm × 0.8 cm × 1.4 cm oval-shaped hypoechoic with center hyperechogenicity in the left lobe.

CDFI: Blood flow signal could be detected in the abnormal echoic wall. Star-spotted blood flow signals could be seen in the oval-shaped hypoechoic nodule.

Sonographic indicates

Multiple fluid-containing mass lesions in the thyroid gland: consider cystic adenoma

Multiple lymphadenopathy in the bilateral neck

Fig. 3.4 Sonographic report of Case 9 (2016-04-22). A 41-year-old male patient presented with a 3.5 cm × 1.5 cm mixed cystic solid nodule in the left lobe on ultrasound

Ultrasonic images:

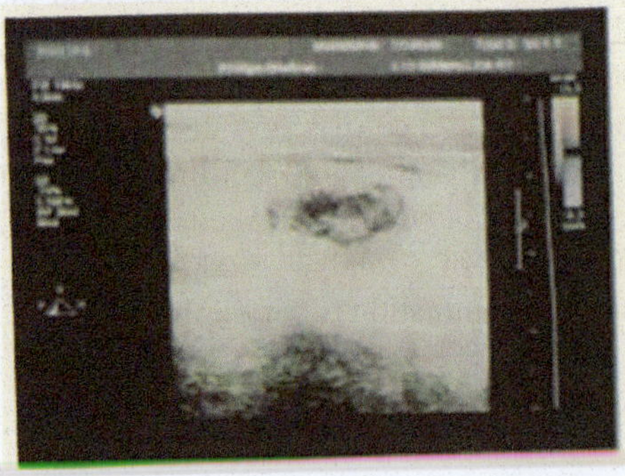

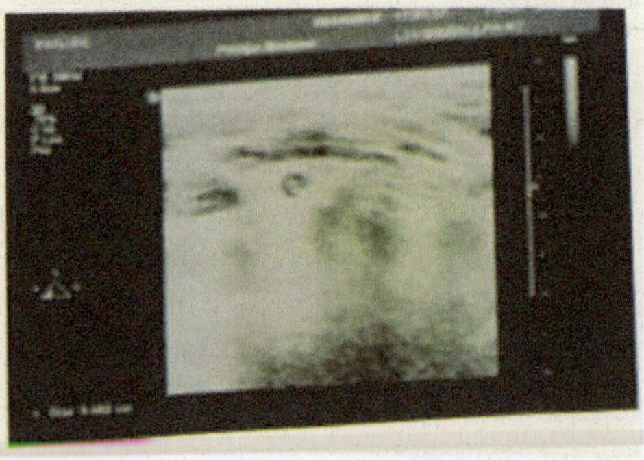

Sonographic findings:

Left lobe: 5.8 cm × 1.8 cm × 1.7 cm;

Right lobe: 5.3 cm × 1.8 cm × 1.8 cm;

Isthmus: anteroposterior diameter is 0.2 cm.

The shape of the thyroid gland was regular. The echogenicity of parenchyma is uneven. A 1.8 cm × 1.3 cm × 1.1cm irregular clumpy hypoechogenicity with sheet hyperechogenicity inside could be detected in the left lobe. A 0.5 cm × 0.4 cm × 0.4 cm irregular clumpy hypoechogenicity with sheet hyperechogenicity inside could be detected in the inferior right lobe.

Bilateral ultrasound scan: Several lymph nodes were detected, one of which was 2.3 cm × 0.7 cm × 1.3 cm oval-shaped hypoechoic with center hyperechogenicity in the left lobe.

CDFI: Blood flow signal could not be detected in the abnormal echoic wall. Star-spotted blood flow signals could be seen in the oval-shaped hypoechoic nodule.

Sonographic indicates

Multiple solid heterogeneous masses in the bilateral lobes (TI-RADS 4a)

Multiple lymphadenopathy in the bilateral neck

Fig. 3.5 Sonographic report of Case 9 (2018-08-06). The nodule changes from 3.5 cm × 1.5 cm to 1.8 cm × 1.1 cm in size

Ultrasonic images:

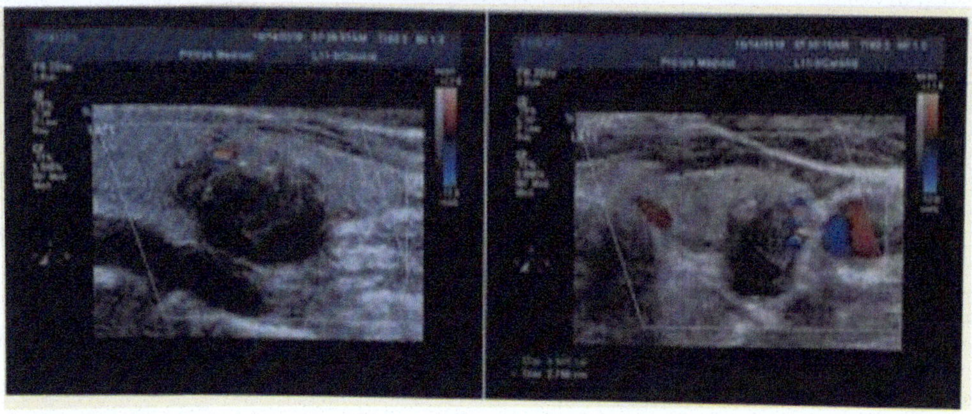

Sonographic findings:

Left lobe: 5.8 cm × 1.8 cm × 1.7 cm;

Right lobe: 5.1 cm × 1.8 cm × 1.9 cm;

Isthmus: anteroposterior diameter is 0.23 cm.

The shape of the thyroid gland was regular. The echogenicity of parenchyma is uneven. A 1.5 cm × 1.9 cm × 1.1cm irregular clumpy hypoechogenicity with sheet hyperechogenicity inside and clear margin could be detected in the inferior left lobe. A 0.2 cm × 0.4 cm × 0.4 cm irregular clumpy very low hypoechogenicity with punctate hyperechogenicity inside and clear margin could be detected in the inferior right lobe.

Bilateral ultrasound scan: Several lymph nodes were detected, one of which was 2.6 cm × 0.8 cm × 1.4 cm oval-shaped hypoechoic with center hyperechogenicity in the left lobe.

CDFI: Blood flow signal could not be detected in the abnormal echoic wall. Blood flow made the round of the hypoechogenicity in the left lobe. Star-spotted blood flow signals could be seen in the oval-shaped hypoechoic nodule.

Sonographic indicates

Uneven solid nodule in the left lobe (TI-RADS 4a)

Multiple lymphadenopathy in the bilateral neck

Fig. 3.6 Sonographic report of Case 9 (2019-10-14). Punctate hyperechogenicity were newly occurred in the left nodule, which might result from the absorption and dehydration of the cystic nodules concomitant with hypoechogenicity and coarse calcifications appear ("zombie" nodules)

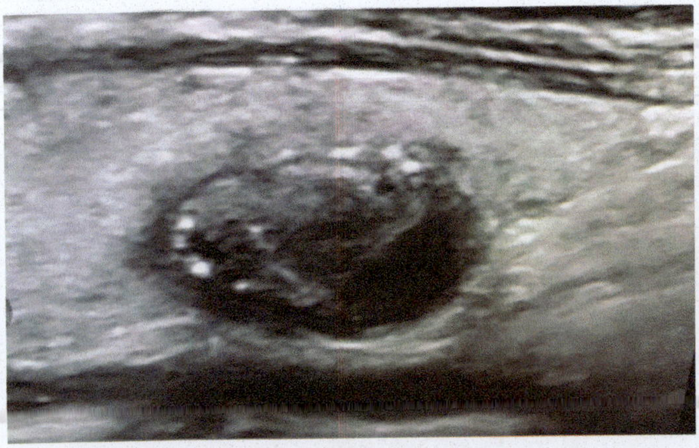

Fig. 3.7 Sonographic imaging of Case 9

Scan the QR code
to watch the ultrasonic video

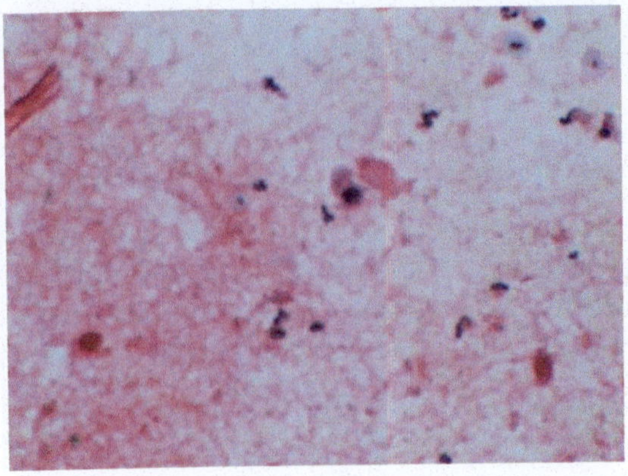

Fig. 3.8 Reports of fine needle aspiration cytology for Case 9. The cytology was a benign tumor. Well-differentiated filtration vesicular epithelial cells were visible

4 Differentiation of Benign and Malignant Nodules in Hashimoto's Thyroiditis

Hashimoto's thyroiditis (HT) is a prevalent autoimmune disease called chronic lymphocytic thyroiditis. It was first described by Hakaru Hashimoto in 1912 and is characterized by the progressive destruction of thyroid follicles. Clinical manifestations are painless thyroid goiter with hypothyroidism (weight gain, fatigue, constipation, mycoedema). HT needs to be diagnosed by serum low T4 and high TSH, accompanied by the presence of thyroglobulin and thyroid peroxidase antibodies. Clinical and serological tests combined with ultrasonography are more sensitive and specific to the diagnosis of HT, but diagnostic criteria are still based on fine needle aspiration biopsy (FNAB) and histological analysis.

The typical clinical manifestations of HT are enlarged, grayish-white, and firm thyroid characterized by interstitial infiltration of hematopoietic monocytes, consisting mainly of lymphocytes, plasma cells, and macrophages (Fig. 4.1). The interstitium becomes degrees of fibrosis, and part of the thyroid cells atrophy, surrounded by small follicles containing small amounts of colloid. In other areas, thyroid cells become larger and thicker, forming a distinctive appearance called Hurthle cells. Hurthle cells are thyroid cells that are enlarged in size, with a chromatin-rich nucleus, and a characteristic cytoplasm that is stained pink by HE due to its presence of mitochondria.

Hashimoto's disease has a variety of sonogram manifestations, and its typical ultrasound images show diffuse enlargement of thyroid glands, increased parenchymal echogenicity, and blood supply. Clear visible hyperechoic fibrous cords with nodular changes are observed in lymph nodes in level VI of the neck (Fig. 4.2). The extent and nature of pathological changes in thyroid nodules vary at different stages, making it challenging to accurately diagnose the nature of thyroid nodules in patients with Hashimoto's thyroiditis who also have nodules. These nodules display complex and diverse changes in imaging characteristics during ultrasound diagnosis. In addition, the insufficient resolution of the ultrasonic instruments and the

G. Wu et al., *Pitfalls in Ultrasound of Thyroid Nodules*,
https://doi.org/10.1007/978-981-19-8873-8_4

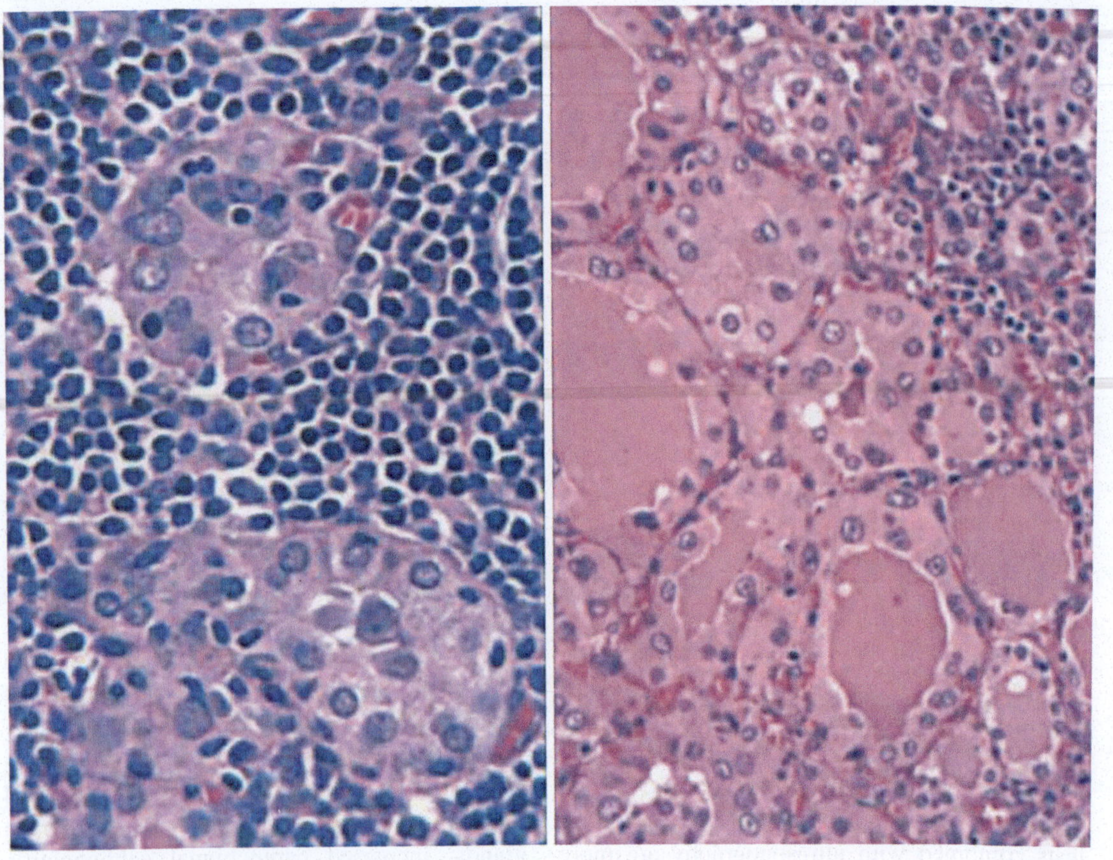

Fig. 4.1 Pathological diagnosis of Hashimoto's thyroiditis. Left image: Two thyroid epithelial follicles that lack any colloid are completely surrounded by lymphocytes and have granular cytoplasm. Right image: eosinophiloid cytoplasm of the filter vesicle epithelium is eosinophilic. The filtration vesicular epithelial cytoplasm is eosinophilic. The nucleus is enlarged and vesicular chromatin, and the nucleoli are prominent and small

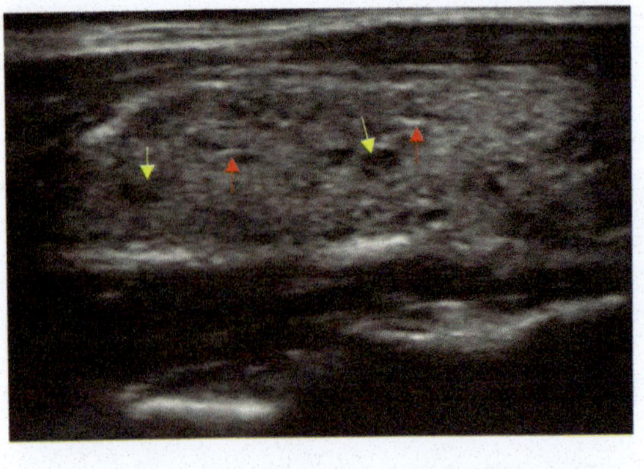

Fig. 4.2 Hashimoto's thyroiditis. In early HT, the size of the gland may be normal with diffuse micronodular changes (yellow arrow) with short-line hyperechogenicity (red arrow) in the parenchyma. Color Doppler Flow Imaging (CDFI) shows diffuse increased blood flow

cognitive and judgment ability of the ultrasound physicians, the diagnostician is easily confused about the benign and malignant nodule sonogram of the thyroid gland in the context of HT. In recent years, some scholars have proposed that papillary thyroid carcinoma (PTC) has a certain relationship with HT. People with Hashimoto's thyroiditis are seven times more likely to have thyroid cancer than healthy people. HT is a risk factor for PTC, and the increase in thyroid-stimulating hormone and persistent stimulation of chronic inflammation caused by HT may lead to an increased incidence of the combination of the two.

Case 10

Clinical information: A 65-year-old female patient was detected with a nodule while health examination. FT3: 5.41 pmol/L (3.21–6.5 pmol/L), FT4: 15.44 pmol/L (10.20–21.88 pmol/L), TSH: 3.44 μU/mL (0.3–4.6 μU/mL), Anti-Tg: 164 U/mL ↑(0–72 U/mL), A-TPO: 3 U/mL (0–16 U/mL).

Ultrasonic information: Fig. 4.3

Preoperative ultrasound evaluation: Fig. 4.4

Gross specimen and pathological diagnosis: Figs. 4.5 and 4.6

Discussion: Misdiagnosis analysis and prevention strategies: The ultrasound features of HT: (1) early stage of HT, the thyroid gland can have no obvious changes or focal echogenicity

Sonographic findings:

Thyroid scan:

Size and shape were normal on thyroid transverse view.

A 0.4 cm × 0.2 cm hypoechoic area could be detected in the inferior right lobe with clear margin and no blood flow.

A 1.1 cm × 0.6 cm hypoechoic area could be detected in the middle left lobe with clear margin, regular shape, and uneven echogenicity inside. Few punctate hyperechogenicity and blood flow could be detected in the left nodule.

Sonographic indicates

A hypo-anechoic area in the right lobe (TI-RADS 3)

A hypoechoic nodule in the left lobe (TI-RADS 4b)

Fig. 4.3 Sonographic report of Case 10

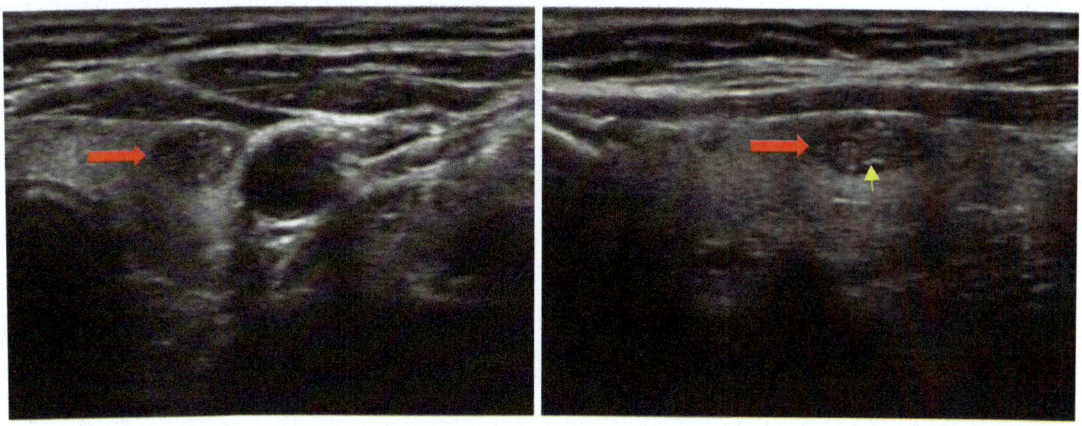

Fig. 4.4 Preoperative ultrasonic reevaluation of Case 10. Hypoechoic nodules were extremely visible in the middle of the left lobe, with a clear margin and punctate hyperechogenicity inside. Changing the direction of the probe, the punctate hyperechogenicity would be extended to a linear hyperechogenicity (yellow arrow). The cross-section of the linear hyperechogenicity can present punctate hyperechogenicity in ultrasound. The probe needs to be rotated in multiple directions to avoid misdiagnosis of the streaked hyperechogenicity as punctate calcification

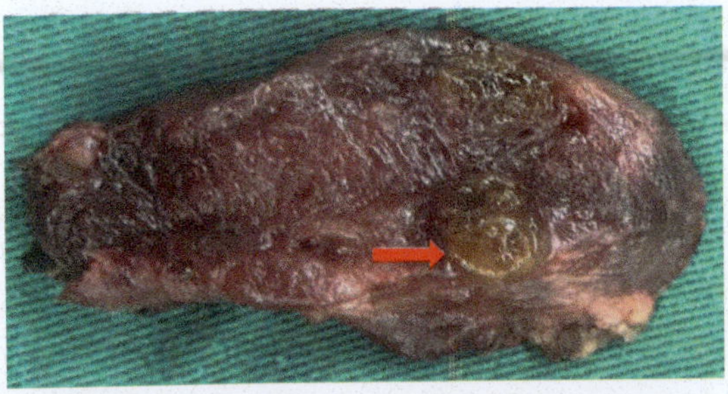

Fig. 4.5 Gross specimen of Case 10. Tough nodules could be palpated in the middle of the left lobe. The nodule was gray-brown and colloid after the incision (red arrows)

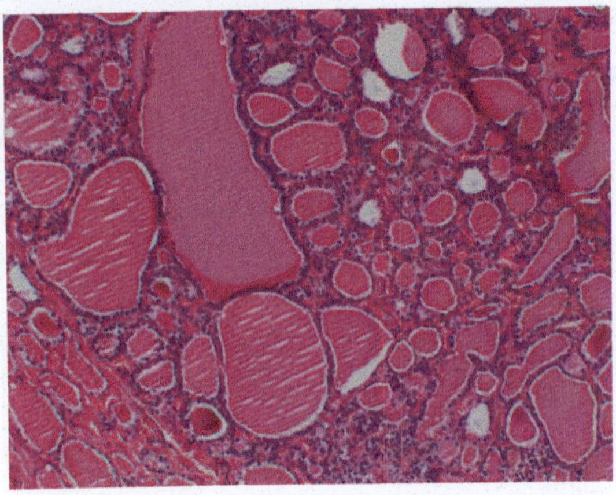

Fig. 4.6 Pathological diagnosis. Hashimoto's thyroiditis

reduction, fine linear hyperechogenicity has not yet formed. (2) Middle and late stages of HT present typical fibrosis change. Diffuse inhomogeneity reduced echogenicity and wide fine-line hyperechogenicity interwoven into a grid can be detected. (3) Advanced stage of HT presents inflammatory nodule formation: single or multiple nodules can be observed in the gland, false nodules (inflammatory nodules) are formed, 1–7 mm in diameter, mostly appearing as hypoechogenicity. (4) Color Doppler blood flow imaging signs: there is no obvious blood flow signal in the bilateral superior thyroid artery in the early stage of HT, the flow rate is normal. The blood flow signal is more abundant in the middle and late stages, or "fire sign," the flow rate increases.

Some acoustic features of thyroid nodules, such as hypoechondria, microcalcification foci, silent halo, aspect ratio imbalance, irregular appearance, and unclear boundaries, are features that suggest malignancy. Punctate hyperechogenicity is not necessarily microcalcifications, and there are two common misdiagnoses: (1) Regarded punctate hyperechogenicity as microcalcifications; (2) neglect the fine linear hyperechogenicity in the nodule, and a multidirectional change probe is required.

Case 11

Clinical information: A 22-year-old female patient was detected with a nodule while health examination. FT3: 4.76 (3.21–6.5 pmol/L), FT4: 18.4 (10.20–21.88 pmol/L), TSH: 2.63 (0.3–4.6 μU/mL), Anti-Tg: 3242 ↑ (0–72 U/mL), A-TPO: 976 ↑ (0–16 U/mL).

Ultrasonic information: Different physicians evaluate the nodule received different reports. The ultrasound resolution affects the ultrasound results to some extent (Figs. 4.7 and 4.8).

Preoperative ultrasound evaluation: Fig. 4.9.

Gross specimen and pathological diagnosis: Figs. 4.10 and 4.11.

Discussion: Misdiagnosis analysis and prevention strategies: Solid hypoechogenicity, ill-defined margin, taller than wide, microcalcification, internal blood flow abundance are important diagnostic indicators for PTC. Malignant thyroid nodules usually present solid hypoechoic and infiltrative growths, usually without a capsule. The malignant nodule has irregular morphology and an ill-defined margin. Calcification in thyroid nodules is usually due to rapid cell growth,

Ultrasonic images:

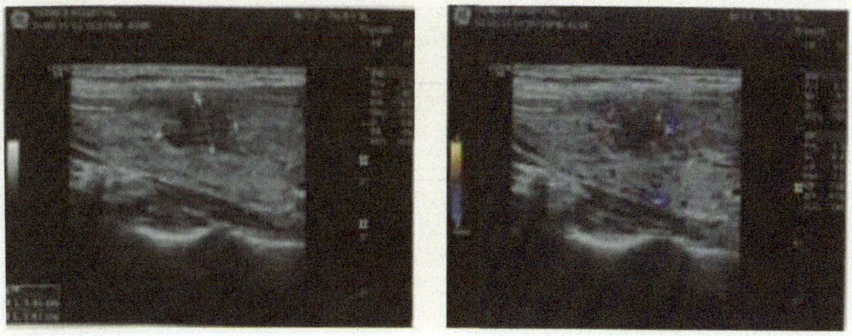

Sonographic findings:

Thyroid scan:

Right lobe: 2.0 cm × 1.9 cm × 8.4 cm.

Left lobe: 2.0 cm × 1.6 cm × 6.8 cm.

Isthmus: anteroposterior diameter is 0.5 cm.

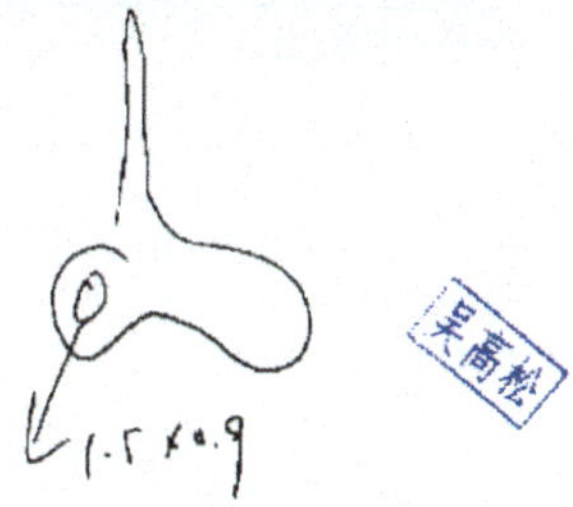

The echogenicity of parenchyma is uneven. A hypoechoic 1.5 cm × 0.9 cm area with clear margin and uneven echogenicity inside in the right lobe. No obvious abnormal echogenicity was detected in the left lobe.

No significantly enlarged lymph nodes were observed in bilateral neck.

CDFI: Blood flow signal could be detected in the hypoechoic area.

Sonographic indicates:

Enlarged thyroid gland and uneven parenchyma

A solid lesion in the right lobe (TI-RADS 3)

Fig. 4.7 Sonographic report of Case 11 (1)

increased vascular and fibrous tissue, and excessive tissue production of calcium salt depositions. Therefore, the clinical value of calcification foci for the diagnosis of thyroid cancer also belongs to a specific index, and microcalcification foci in thyroid malignant nodules are of great significance.

Case 12

Clinical information: A 39-year-old male patient was detected with a nodule while health examination. FT3: 4.78 pmol/L (3.21–6.5 pmol/L), FT4: 15.96 pmol/L (10.20–21.88 pmol/L), TSH: 2.913 μU/mL (0.3–4.6μU/mL), Anti-Tg: 103 U/mL ↑ (0–72 U/mL), A-TPO: 1637 U/mL ↑(0–16 U/mL)

Ultrasonic images:

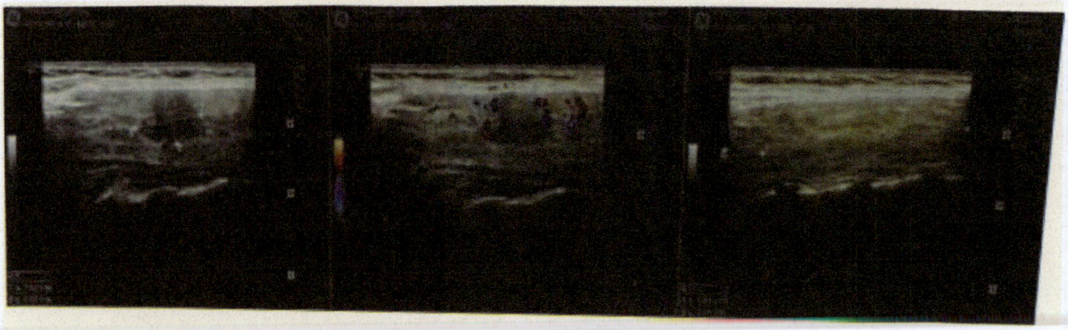

Sonographic findings:

Right lobe: 2.1 cm × 1.8 cm × 6.4 cm.

Left lobe: 1.9 cm × 1.6 cm × 5.9 cm.

Isthmus: anteroposterior diameter is 0.3 cm.

The echogenicity of parenchyma is uneven. A hypoechoic 1.6 cm × 1.1 cm area with irregular shape, ill-defined margin, uneven echogenicity and several punctate hyperechogenicity inside in the right lobe. No obvious abnormal echogenicity was detected in the left lobe.

No significantly enlarged lymph nodes were observed in bilateral neck.

CDFI: Blood flow signal could be detected in the hypoechoic area.

Sonographic indicates:

Diffuse non-uniform enlargement of the thyroid gland (Hashimoto's thyroiditis?)

A solid lesion in the right lobe with microcalcification (TI-RADS 4b)

Fig. 4.8 Sonographic report of Case 11 (2)

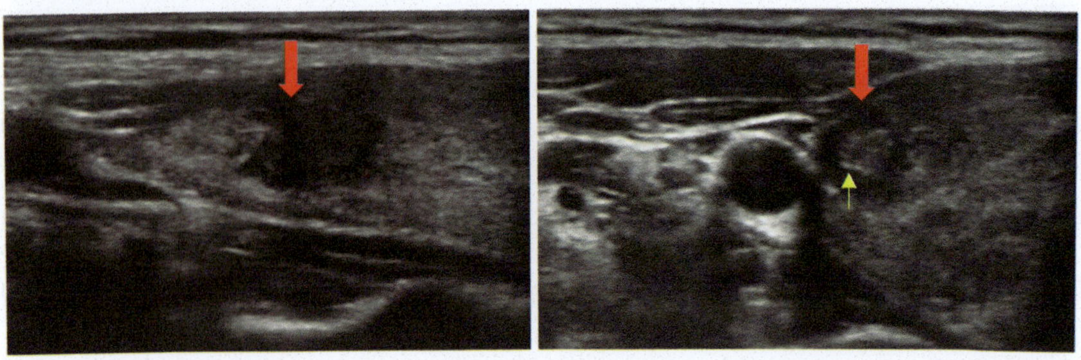

Fig. 4.9 Preoperative ultrasonic reevaluation of Case 11 (2). Irregular shape nodule with punctate hyperechogenicity inside in the right lobe

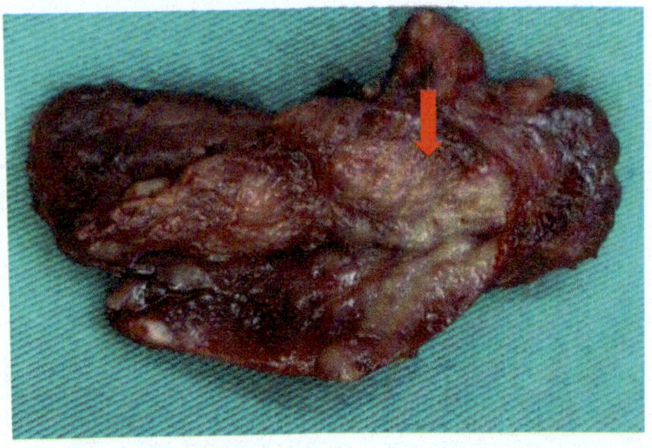

Fig. 4.10 Gross specimen of Case 11. Several gray and white lesions in the right lobe, with ill-defined margin (red arrows)

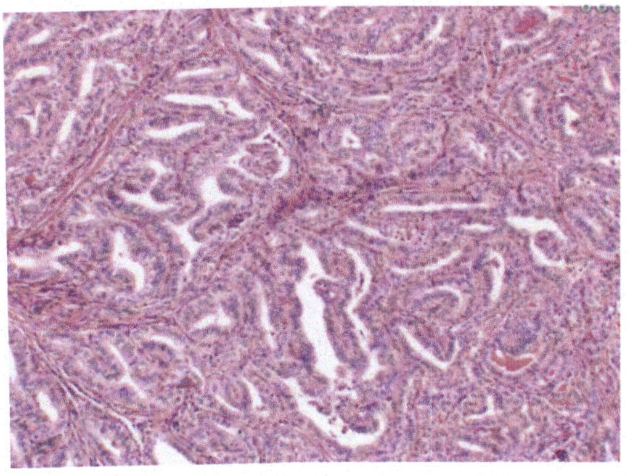

Fig. 4.11 Pathological diagnosis. Papillary thyroid carcinoma

Ultrasonic information: Fig. 4.12

Preoperative ultrasound evaluation: Fig. 4.13

Gross specimen and pathological diagnosis: Figs. 4.14, 4.15, 4.16, 4.17, and 4.18

Discussion: Misdiagnosis analysis and prevention strategies: Kim et al. applied taller-than-wide nodule as the evaluation of thyroid cancer, pointing out this diagnostic method is not sensitive, but highly specific. For thyroid carcinoma concomitant with Hashimoto's thyroiditis, there are different degrees of follicular cell destruction and disappearance, fibrosis, and lymphatic cell infiltration, resulting in irregular growth of thyroid nodules, which is easily confused with the growth mode of increased anteroposterior diameter of malignant thyroid nodules. However, if there are common malignant features of thyroid cancer, it is recommended to perform fine needle aspiration cytology.

Case 13

Clinical information: A 60-year-old female patient presented with cervical mass for four years. Specialized physical examination: Diffuse enlargement of the bilateral thyroid gland. Tough nodules about 2.5 cm in the left and right thyroid lobes could be palpated, which moves up and down along with swallowing.

FT3: 4.66 pmol/L (3.21–6.5 pmol/L), FT4: 14.16 pmol/L (10.20–21.88 pmol/L), TSH: 1.11 μU/mL (0.3–4.6 μU/mL), Anti-Tg: 228 U/mL ↑ (0–72 U/mL), A-TPO: 2 U/mL (0–16 U/mL).

Ultrasonic information: Multiple nodules are visible in the bilateral lobes, with hyperechoic foci visible in the very low hypoechoic area in the right lobe (Fig. 4.19).

Preoperative ultrasound evaluation: Ultrasound showing hyperechoic foci is more likely to be considered for malnutrition calcification. Thyroid calcification refers to the deposition of calcium in the nodule. When the acoustic impedance of the reflective interface is large, it is manifested in various forms of hyperechogenicity on ultrasound, with or without sound and acoustic shadowing. Malnutrition calcification is due to the rapid growth of cancer cells, tissue proliferation, degeneration, calcium salt deposition, resulting in calcification (Fig. 4.20).

Gross specimen and pathological diagnosis: Figs. 4.21 and 4.22

Discussion: Misdiagnosis analysis and prevention strategies: The calcification of PTC concomitant with HT is common and diverse, calcification occurs in the background of HT, whether microcalcification, coarse calcification, or isolated calcification suggests a malignant risk, so careful observation of calcification is helpful to improve the diagnostic rate of PTC in HT background. Ohmori et al. found that dense

Ultrasonic images:

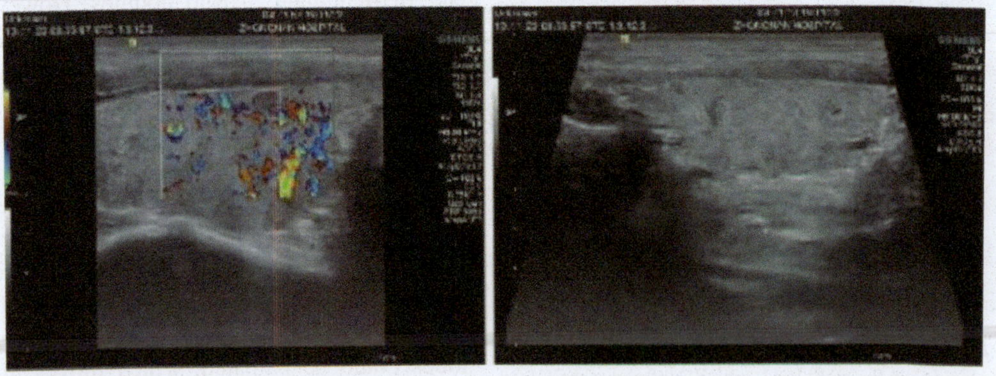

Sonographic findings:

Thyroid scan

Right lobe: 4.5 cm × 1.8 cm × 2.0 cm.

Left lobe: 3.7 cm × 1.5 cm × 1.8 cm.

Isthmus: anteroposterior diameter is 0.25 cm.

Size and shape were normal on thyroid transverse view. The echogenicity of parenchyma is hypoechoic and uneven.

A hypoechoic 0.2 cm × 0.3 cm area with ill-defined margin and uneven echogenicity in the inferior left lobe. The taller than wide nodule contained blood flow sign inside.

A hypoechoic 0.3 cm × 0.4 cm area with ill-defined margin and uneven echogenicity in the inferior left lobe. The taller than wide nodule did not detect blood flow sign inside.

CDFI: Blood flow sign increased in the thyroid parenchyma.

Sonographic indicates:

Diffuse lesions of the thyroid gland

A hypoechoic area in the right lobe (TI-RADS 4a)

A hypoechoic area in the left lobe (TI-RADS 4a, tend to be benign)

Fig. 4.12 Sonographic report of Case 12

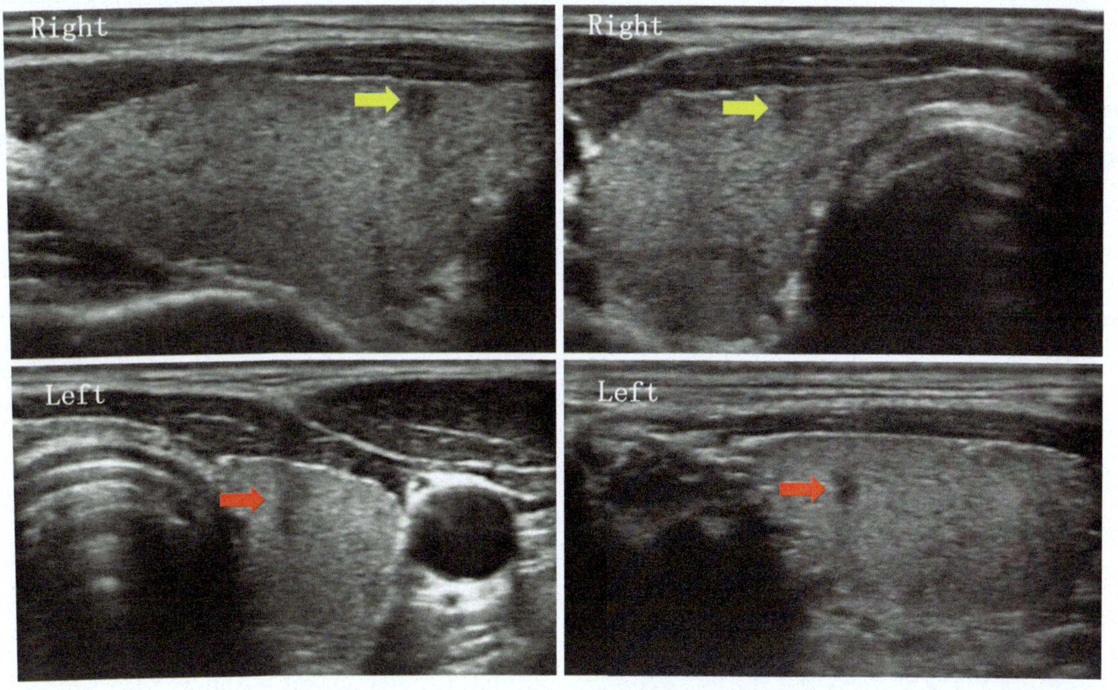

Fig. 4.13 Preoperative ultrasonic reevaluation of Case 12. The common feature of bilateral nodules is taller than wide. In view of the relatively small nodules, the decreased echogenicity of the glands is not easily distinguished from Hashimoto's thyroiditis

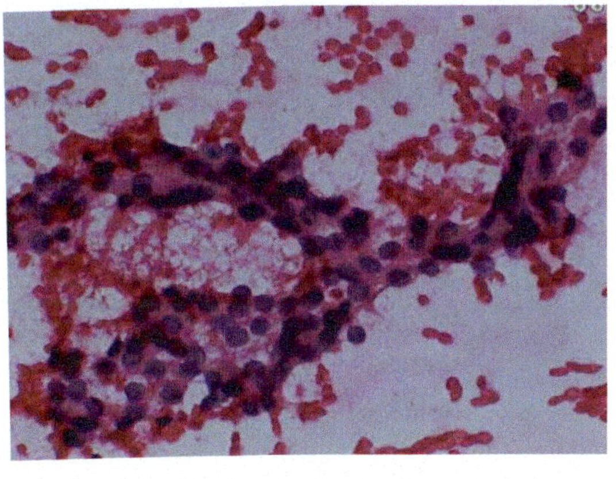

Fig. 4.14 Pathological diagnosis of Case 12 (1)

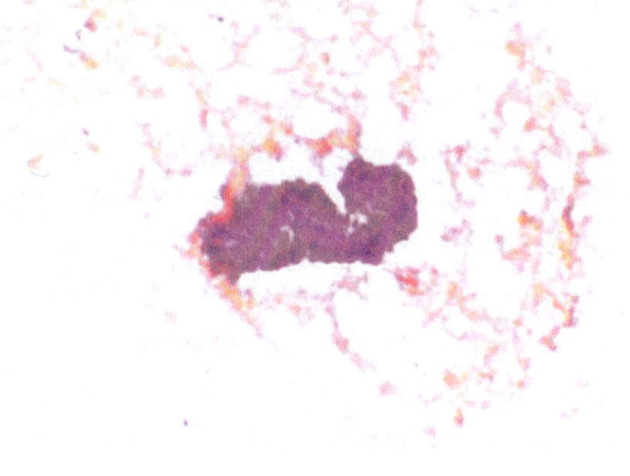

Fig. 4.15 Pathological diagnosis of Case 12 (2)

Results of FNAC:

1. (smear of cells from the left thyroid lobe combined with liquid-based cytology)

Papillary thyroid carcinoma was suspected.

Abnormal follicular epithelial cells and nuclear grooves were observed.

2. (smear of cells from the right thyroid lobe combined with liquid-based cytology)

Papillary thyroid carcinoma.

Anormal follicular epithelial cells, nuclear grooves and intranuclear pseudoinclusions were observed.

Fig. 4.16 Pathological diagnosis of Case 12 (3)

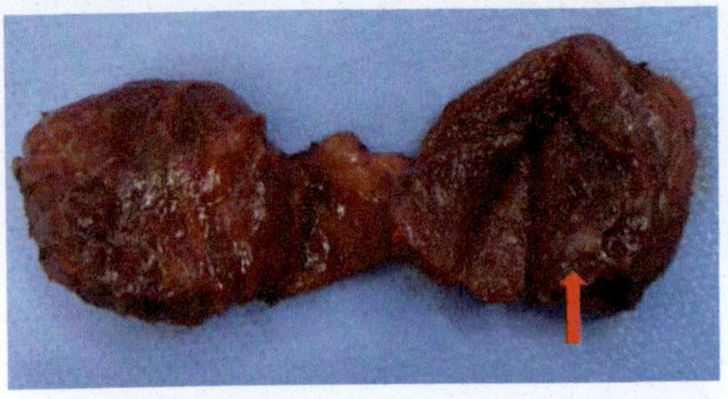

Fig. 4.17 Gross specimen of case 12. A 0.2-cm gray-white nodule in the left lobe (red arrows)

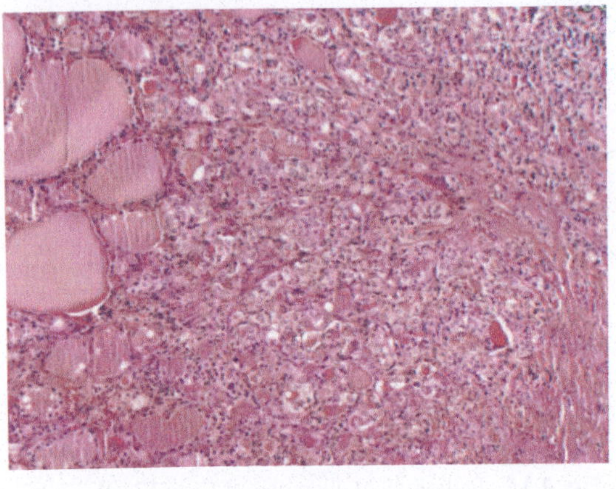

Fig. 4.18 Pathological diagnosis of Case 12 Bilateral papillary thyroid microcarcinoma

calcification foci were more often occurred in the papillary thyroid cancer patients concomitant with HT, while psammoma bodies were rare. Therefore, attention should be paid to calcification observed in the HT background nodules.

Case 14

Clinical information: A 66-year-old female patient presented with thyroid nodule for one year. FT3: 5.21 pmol/L (3.21–6.5 pmol/L), FT4: 12.36 pmol/L (10.20–21.88 pmol/L), TSH: 3.41 μU/mL (0.3–4.6 μU/mL), Anti-Tg: 345 U/mL ↑ (0–72 U/mL), A-TPO: 763 U/mL ↑ (0–16 U/mL).

Ultrasonic information: Ultrasounds in different institutions presented hypoechoic nodules on the left dorsal lobe, with hyperechoic inside (Figs. 4.23 and 4.24).

Preoperative ultrasound evaluation: Fig. 4.25

Gross specimen and pathological diagnosis: Figs. 4.26, 4.27, and 4.28

Discussion: Misdiagnosis analysis and prevention strategies: Diffuse reduced echogenicity of HT were detected, diffuse reduction of the degree of bilateral thyroid echogenicity with different degrees, bilateral lobes with irregular shape and unclear margin, and hyperechogenicity of varying thickness and thickness, irregular fibrous cords; the pathological basis for the localization of the thyroid gland, extensive or nodular hypoechondria is that the number of inflammatory cells that appear in the thyroid tissue are fociform or scattered infiltration, and even the formation of lymphatic follicles of different sizes and the obvious hair growth heart. In the context of HT, solid hypoechogenicity, unclear margin, and irregular morphological patterns are all screening indicators with good sensitivity; however, the specificity of ultrasound diagnosis is

Sonographic findings:

Thyroid scan

Left lobe: 5.7 cm × 2.0 cm × 1.6 cm.

Right lobe: 6.1 cm × 1.8 cm × 2.0 cm.

Isthmus: anteroposterior diameter is 0.67 cm.

Size and shape were normal on thyroid transverse view. The echogenicity of parenchyma is hypoechoic and uneven, with patchy hypoechoic foci inside.

Left lobe: A hypoechoic 1.83 cm × 0.46 cm nodule with ill-defined margin, irregular shape, and uneven echogenicity inside in the superior left lobe. A sightly low hypoechoic 2.47 cm × 1.25 cm nodule with ill-defined margin, and uneven echogenicity inside in the inferior left lobe.

Right lobe: Several hypoechoic foci with ill-defined margin and uneven echogenicity inside in the right lobe, one of which was 0.49 cm × 0.28 cm in size. A hypoechoic 0.44 cm × 0.40 cm nodule with ill-defined margin, uneven echogenicity and hyperechoic foci inside in the inferior right lobe.

CDFI: Blood flow sign increased in the thyroid parenchyma. Colored blood flow signals were observed in the hypoechoic and sightly low hypoechoic nodules in the left lobe. No obvious colored blood flow signals were observed in the hypoechoic nodule in the right lobe.

Sonographic indicates:

Diffuse lesions of the thyroid gland

A hypoechoic area in the inferior right lobe with calcification (TI-RADS 4a)

Hypoechoic areas in the bilateral lobes (TI-RADS 3)

Sightly low hypoechoic nodule in the left lobe (TI-RADS 3)

Fig. 4.19 Sonographic report of Case 13

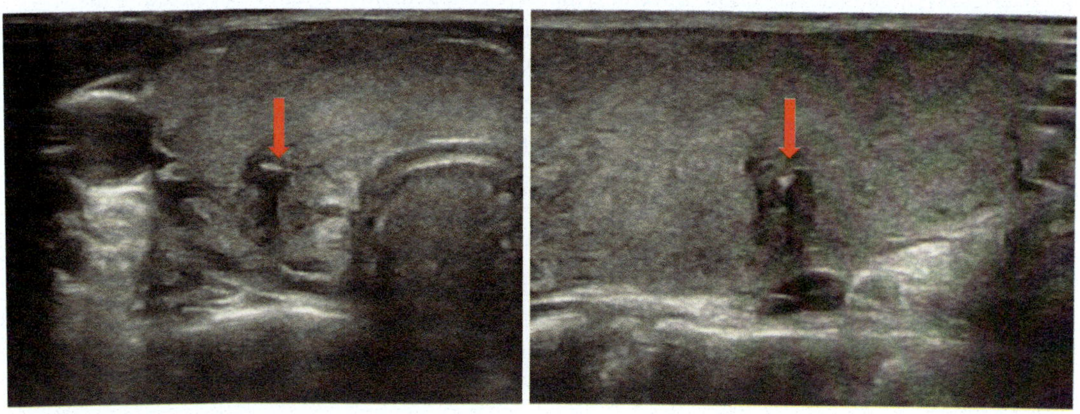

Fig. 4.20 Preoperative ultrasonic reevaluation of Case 13

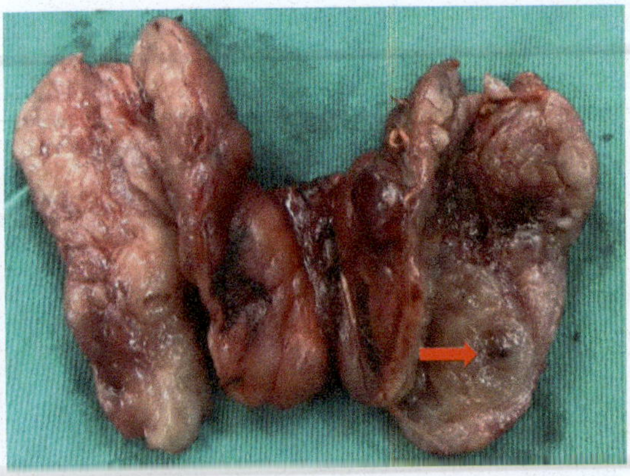

Fig. 4.21 Gross specimen of Case 13. The cross section was gray-red and gray-brown in the bilateral lobes, part of which was gray and ill-defined margin with surrounding tissue (red arrows)

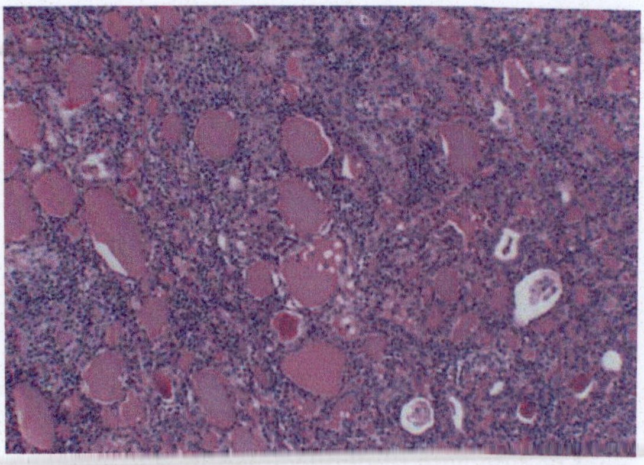

Fig. 4.22 Pathological diagnosis. Bilateral Hashimoto's thyroiditis

Ultrasonic images:

Thyroid scan

Left lobe: 31.3 mm × 12.6 mm × 18.8 mm.

Right lobe: 42.7 mm × 18.4 mm × 19.2 mm.

Isthmus: anteroposterior diameter is 6.3 mm.

The shape of the thyroid gland was normal. Several hypoechoic nodules vary in size were detected in left lobe, one of which was taller than wide 5.5 mm × 5.1 mm nodule in the inferior dorsal gland with regular shape and uneven echogenicity inside. A 2.2 mm× 2.2 mm hyperechoic foci and a 6.8 cm × 4.4 cm anechoic nodule in the middle of left lobe could be observed.

CDFI: No blood flow sign increased in the nodules.

Cervical lymph node detection: Several lymphatic echogenicities could be detected in the bilateral levels I, II, III with normal shape. The lymph nodes were taller than wide, the cortical medulla was clearly demarcated and the lymphatic portal was visible. A 4.8 mm× 3.0 mm enlarged lymph node in left level II and a 5.4 mm 3.1 mm in right level II.

CDFI: No blood flow sign increased in the lymph nodes.

Sonographic indicates:

Uneven thyroid texture (Hashimoto thyroiditis)

Solid nodules in the bilateral lobes (TI-RADS 3)

Cystic nodule in the left lobe (TI-RADS 2)

Solid nodule in the left lobe with coarse calcification (taller than wide TI-RADS 4a)

Fig. 4.23 Sonographic report of Case 14 (1)

Sonographic findings:

Thyroid scan

Part of the left lobe was behind the clavicle and was difficult to observe.

Left lobe: 6.1 cm × 1.9 cm × 1.6 cm.

Right lobe: 6.3 cm × 2.0 cm × 1.9 cm.

Isthmus: anteroposterior diameter is 0.55 cm.

The shape of the thyroid gland was normal. The echogenicity of parenchyma is sightly hypoechoic and uneven. Several patchy hypoechoic areas and striped hyperechoic foci were detected.

Several anechoic areas could be observed in the left lobe with clear margin and hyperechogenicity behind, one of which was a 0.8 cm × 0.4 cm nodule.

A 0.6 cm × 0.5 cm hyperechoic nodule in the superior dorsal of left lobe could be observed with ill-defined margin and uneven echogenicity inside. A 0.4 cm × 0.3 cm hyperechoic foci were seen inside.

CDFI: No blood flow sign increased in the aforementioned nodules.

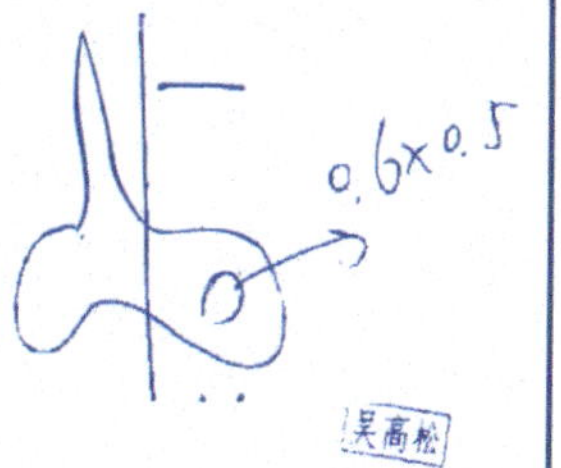

Sonographic indicates:

Diffuse heterogeneous lesions of the thyroid (Hashimoto thyroiditis?)

Anechoic areas in the left lobe (cyst?)

Hypoechoic nodule in the left lobe with calcification (TI-RADS 4a)

Fig. 4.24 Sonographic report of Case 14 (2)

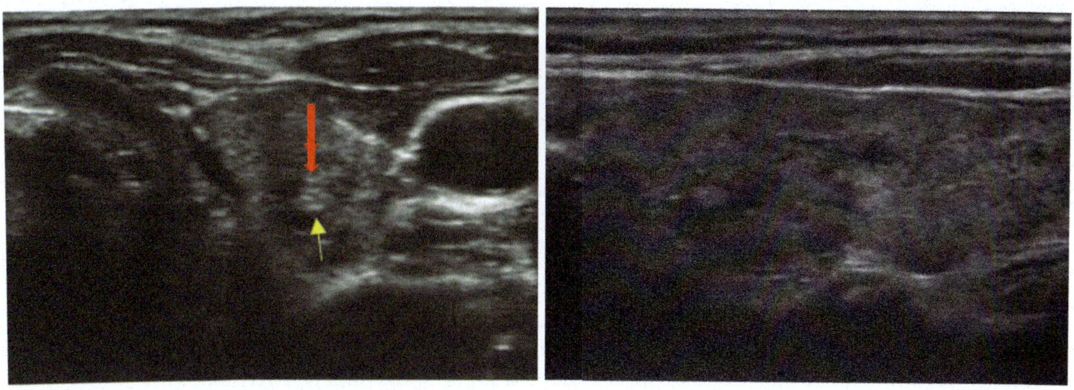

Fig. 4.25 Preoperative ultrasonic reevaluation of Case 14

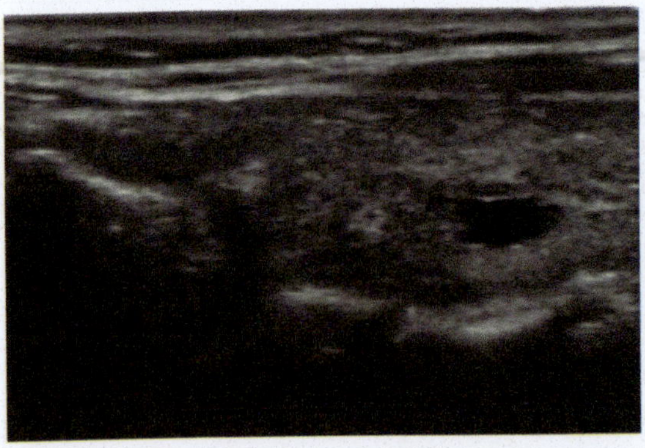

Fig. 4.26 Sonographic report of Case 14 (3)

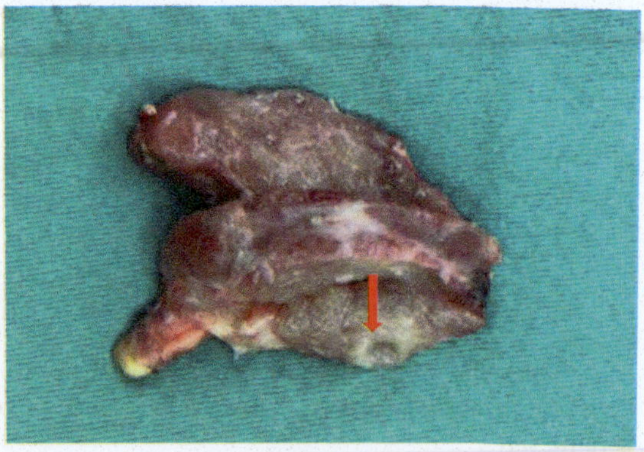

Fig. 4.27 Gross specimen of Case 14

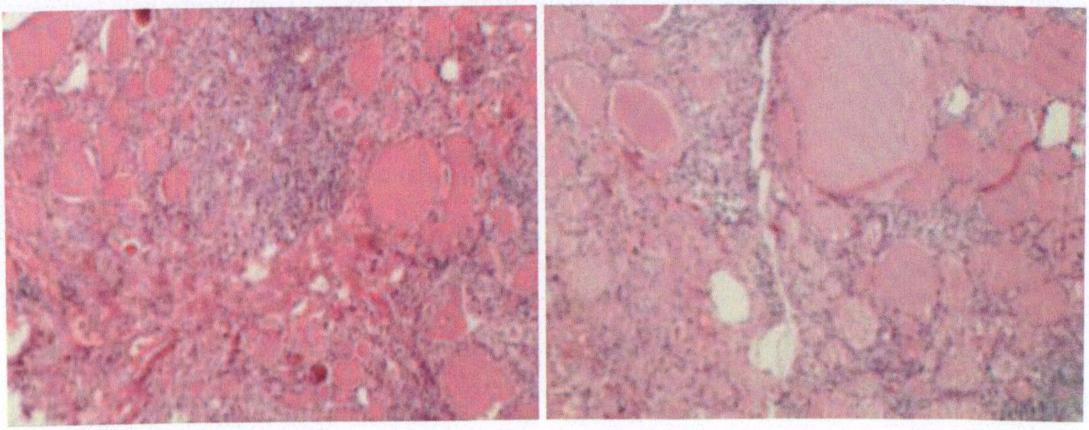

Fig. 4.28 Pathological diagnosis. (Left thyroid) Hashimoto's thyroiditis with local follicular epithelial squamous epithelial metaplasia. Immunohistochemistry: CD56 (+), CK19 (+), Galectin-3 (−), HBME-1 (−), TPO (+), TTF-1 (+), P40 (+), P63 (+)

low, and only the taller than wide is an ideal specificity indicator. Therefore, ultrasound has a high rate of misdiagnosis of benign nodules in the context of HT, and for patients with thyroid nodules concomitant with HT who have a tendency to diagnose malignancy in ultrasound, it should be highly recommended that fine needle aspiration cytology be performed to avoid unnecessary surgical treatment.

Case 15

Clinical information: A 53-year-old female patient was detected with a nodule while health examination for one week. FT3: 5.62 pmol/L (3.21–6.5 pmol/L), FT4: 12.69 pmol/L (10.20–21.88 pmol/L), TSH: 1.4 μU/mL (0.3–4.6 μU/mL), Anti-Tg: 630 U/mL ↑(0–72 U/mL), A-TPO: 19 U/mL ↑ (0–16 U/mL).

Ultrasonic information: A taller-than-wide nodule in the superior left lobe (Fig. 4.29).

Preoperative ultrasound evaluation: Fig. 4.30

Gross specimen and pathological diagnosis: Figs. 4.31 and 4.32

Discussion: Misdiagnosis analysis and prevention strategies: The ultrasound nodules in Case 12 and Case 15 are similarly described, but

Sonographic findings:

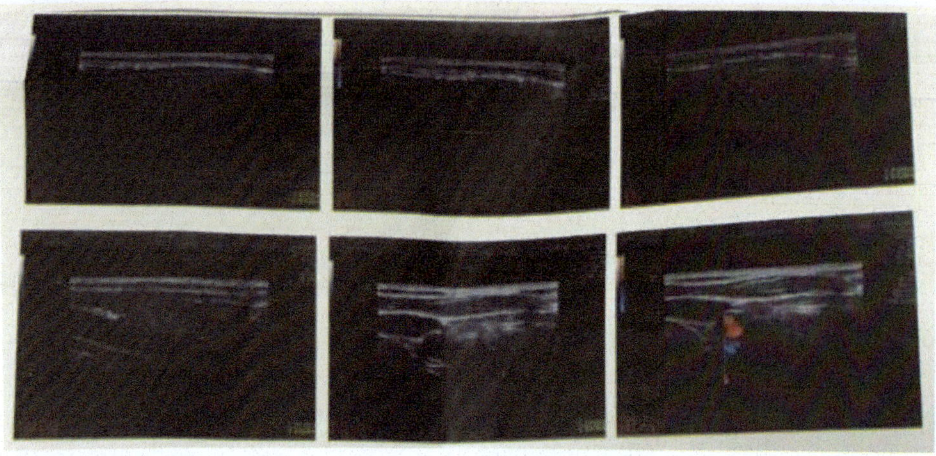

Apply for examination: Thyroid superficial lymph nodes / neck

Sonographic findings:

The shape of the thyroid gland was sightly enlarged. The echogenicity of parenchyma is uneven with several cystic, solid and mixed nodule inside, one of which was a 2.9 mm × 4.4 mm solid hypoechoic nodule in the superior left lobe with ill-defined margin and taller than wide. A 5.2 mm× 2.9 mm mixed nodule mainly in solid with clear margin in the middle inferior left lobe and a 3.3 mm× 2.4 mm mixed nodule in the middle inferior right lobe with clear margin were observed. A hypo-anechoic 8.3 cm × 7.6 cm nodule in the inferior dorsal right lobe with clear margin was detected.

CDFI: No abnormal blood flow signal could be detected in the thyroid and the nodules.

Abnormal echogenicity was detected in bilateral lymph nodes. Lymph nodes in both left and level II were seen, 11.1 mm × 5.2 mm and 21.2 mm × 6.9 mm in size, respectively.

Sonographic indicates:

A solid hypoechoic nodule in the superior left lobe with taller than wide and ill-defined margin

Fig. 4.29 Sonographic report of Case 15

the histological type in Case 12 is papillary thyroid carcinoma, while the histological type in Case 15 is chronic lymphocytic thyroiditis, so the growth pattern of thyroid nodules in patients with Hashimoto's thyroiditis and papillary thyroid carcinoma is irregular, which is easily confused with the growth pattern of increased anterior and posterior diameter of malignant thyroid nodules. Fine needle aspiration cytology was recommended to diagnose.

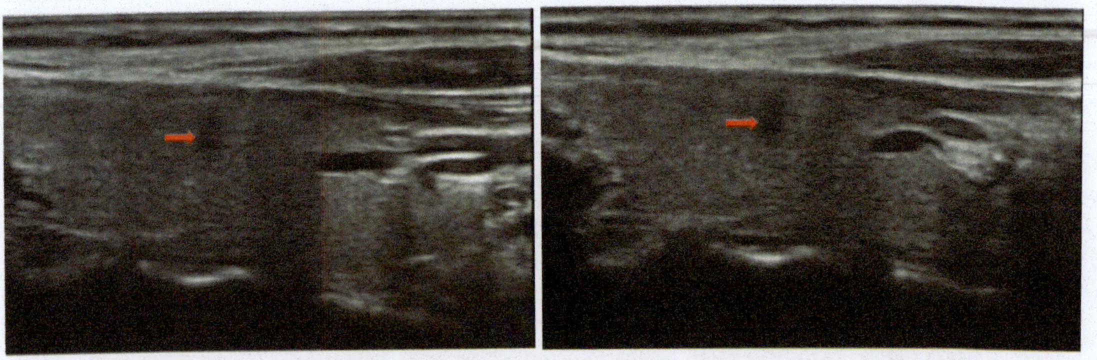

Fig. 4.30 Preoperative ultrasonic reevaluation of Case 15

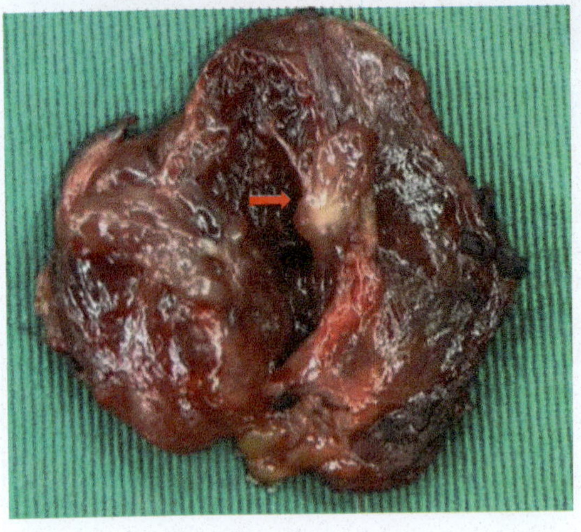

Fig. 4.31 Gross specimen of Case 15. The cut surface is grayish-brown without obvious nodules

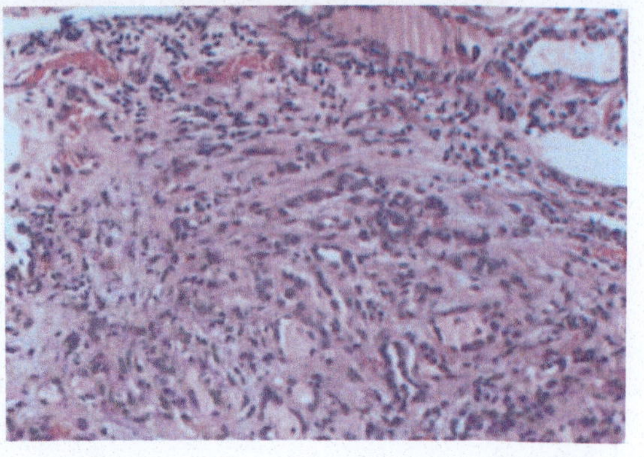

Fig. 4.32 Pathological diagnosis (left) chronic lymphocytic thyroiditis

Further Readings

Caturegli P, De Remigis A, Rose NR. Hashimoto thyroiditis: clinical and diagnostic criteria. Autoimmun Rev. 2014;13(4):391–7.

Caturegli P, Ruggere C. Karl Hurthle! Now, who was he? Thyroid. 2005;15:121–3.

Friedman M, Shimaoka K, Rao U, et al. Diagnosis of chronic lymphocytic thyroiditis (nodular presentation) by needle aspiration. Acta Cytol. 1981;25(5):513–22.

Hashimoto H. Zur Kenntus der Lymphomatosen veranderung der Schildruse (Struma Lymphomatosa). Arch Kin Chir. 1912;97:219.

Kim EK, Park CS, Chung WY, et al. New sonographic criteria for recommending fine-needle aspiration biopsy of nonpalpable solid nodules of the thyroid. AJR Am J Roentgenol. 2002;178(3):687–91.

Li Y, Nishihara E, Kakudo K. Hashimoto's thyroiditis: old concepts and new insights. Curr Opin Rheumatol. 2011;23(1):102–7.

Li Q, Zhang J, Zou X, et al. Ultrasonography characteristics in diagnosis of thyroid microcarcinoma. Chin J Ultrasound. 2009;25(10):940–3.

Nordmeyer JP, Shafeh TA, Heckmann C. Thyroid sonography in autoimmune thyroiditis. A prospective study on 123 patients. Acta Endocrinol (Copenh). 1990;122(3):391–5.

Ohmori N, Miyakawa M, Ohmori K, et al. Ultrasonographic findings of papillary thyroid carcinoma with Hashimoto's thyroiditis. Intern Med, 2007 , 46(9):547-550.

Wang X, Zheng K, Huang M. Clinicopathological and ultrasonographic characteristics of papillary thyroid carcinoma combined with Hashimoto's thyroiditis. Chin J Med Imaging. 2018;26(10):747–51.

Yao L, Dong Y. Diagnostic value of color Doppler ultrasound combined CT examination on nodular goiter complicated with thyroid cancer. J Med Imaging. 2019;29(2):323–6.

Zhang D, Li Y, Meng Y, Zhai L, Xing J. Ultrasound and pathology analysis of thyroid nodular lesions with Hashimoto's thyroiditis. Chin J Med Ultrasound. 2014;11(8):46–51.

5 Disappearance of Thyroid Nodules

Thyroid ultrasonography should routinely include cervical lymph node examinations. High-resolution ultrasound is equipped with high sensitivity, high specificity, and high accuracy to differentiate benign and malignant lymph nodes, and plays an important role in the management of thyroid malignant tumors. What makes surgeons confused is the absence of lymphatic hilum and disappearance of cutaneous medulla in ultrasound reports.

The normal lymph node structure consists of a central hyperechoic hilum and a peripheral hypoechoic cortex, and the hilum includes adipose tissues and blood vessels (Fig. 5.1). Lymph nodes' shape and their aspect ratios (elliptic or spherical), cortical echogenicity and shape; position and shape (centralization, eccentricity, deformation, disappearance) of medullas; internal echogenicity (with or without calcifications and liquefactions); vascular pattern (no blood flows, lymphatic hilar blood flows, central blood flows, peripheral blood flows or mixed blood flows); boundaries, performances of fusion were observed.

Ultrasonographic features of suspected malignant lymph nodes include microcalcifications

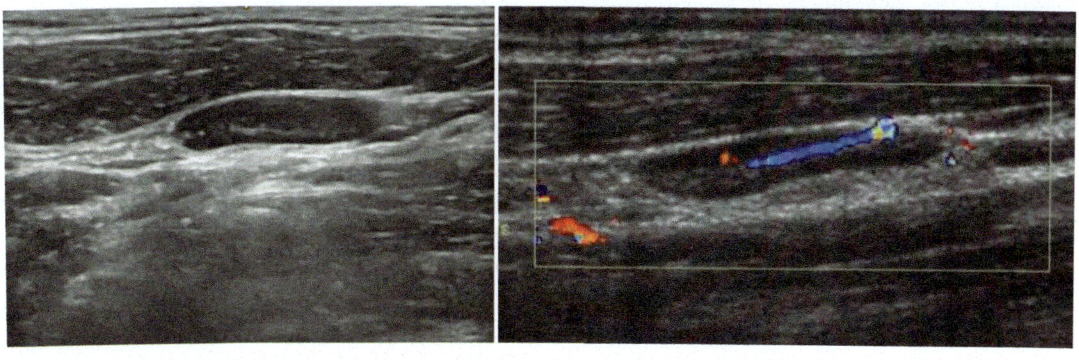

Fig. 5.1 Normal lymph nodes present as hypoechoic oval structure, a central linear hyperechogenicity for the lymphatic hilum, blood flow enters through the lymph node hilum and extends inward along the long axis, there is no blood flow signal around the periphery, and the length/short ratio is >2

Supplementary Information The online version contains supplementary material available at https://doi.org/10.1007/978-981-19-8873-8_5.

G. Wu et al., *Pitfalls in Ultrasound of Thyroid Nodules*,
https://doi.org/10.1007/978-981-19-8873-8_5

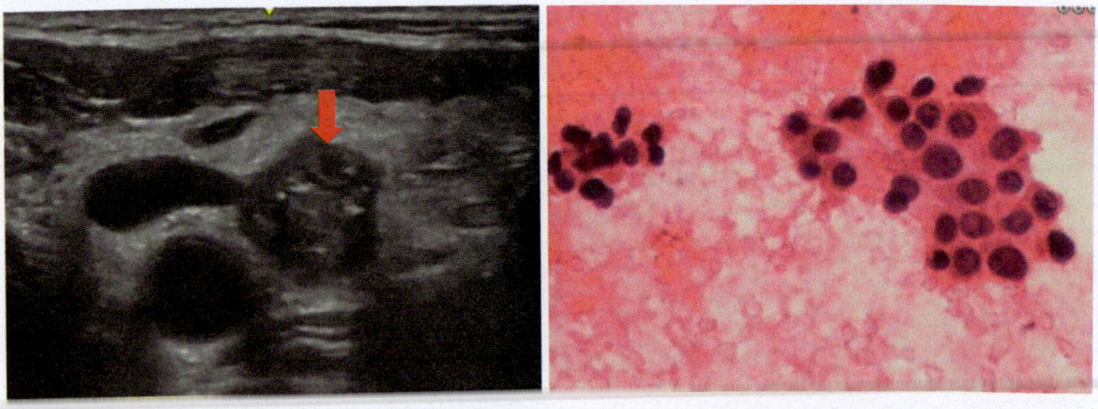

Fig. 5.2 Punctate hyperechogenicity occurred in the lymph nodes, suspected malignancy, and fine needle aspiration cytology show metastatic papillary thyroid carcinoma

(Fig. 5.2), cystic changes, mass hyperechogenicity, enlarged anterior and posterior diameter of lymph nodes, and peripheral blood flows. Lymph node sizes should not be the standard for differentiating benign lymph nodes from malignant ones. Benign lymph nodes are flat in shape with a length/short ratio exceeding 2. Malignant lymph nodes are rounder in shape with a length/short ratio of less than 2. Steinkamp et al. found that the critical value of length/short ratio in the differential diagnosis of benign and malignant cervical lymph nodes was 2, and the accuracy reaches 95%. Leboulleux et al. subsequently found that this threshold only has a sensitivity of 46% and a specificity of 64% (Table 5.1).

Disappearance of lymphatic hilum may be caused by tumor invasion blocking lymphatic reflux. Not all hilum of lymph nodes can be seen in ultrasound, and the specificity of hilums' absence for identifying malignancy is only 29%. Therefore, lymph nodes with sonographic findings of lymphatic hilum are often benign, but the absence of lymphatic hilum structure does not necessarily refer to metastasis. Any calcification found in the lymph nodes, whether microcalcification or irregular calcification with acoustic shadowing, is a strong indication of malignancy. Cystic necrosis in lymph nodes is also a specific sign of malignancy (but can also be detected in lymph node tuberculosis).

Table 5.1 Sensitivity and specificity of ultrasound in diagnosing different characteristic performances of thyroid nodules

Characteristic performances	Sensitivity (%)	Specificity (%)
Short diameter > 0.5 cm	61	96
long diameter > 1 cm	68	75
length/short ratio < 2	46	64
No hyperechoic lymphatic hilum is observed	100	29
Hypoechoic change	39	18
Punctate hyperechogenicity (calcification)	46	100
Cystic degeneration	11	100
Disturbances in peripheral blood flow signals	86	82

Case 16

Clinical information: A 70-year-old male patient received a neck ultrasound reexamination after medullary thyroid cancer surgery for two years. Lymph nodes in levels III and IV of the left neck were abnormal. CEA: 41.13 ng/mL↑(≤ 5.0 ng/mL), calcitonin: 1823 pg/mL ↑(<100 pg/mL).

Ultrasonic information: Shape of lymph nodes in levels III and IV was abnormal Lymph node puncture, eluent CEA, and calcitonin measurement were recommended. The 2015 American Thyroid Association (ATA) Guidelines for the Diagnosis and Treatment of Thyroid Nodules and Thyroid Adenocarcinoma in Adults states that if the minimum diameter of suspected lymph nodes is > 8–10 mm, ultrasound-guided FNA should be performed to determine the surgical modalities after a definitive diagnosis (Fig. 5.3).

Preoperative ultrasound evaluation: Figs. 5.4 and 5.5

Pathological diagnosis: Fig. 5.6

Sonographic findings:

Several oval lymphatic echogenicity were detected in the level II, VI of right neck with normal shape and clear cortical medullary margin, one of which were 1.2 cm × 0.4 cm and 1.0 cm× 0.6 cm in level II and VI, respectively.

Several oval lymphatic echogenicity were detected in the level II of left neck with normal shape and clear cortical medullary margin, one of which were 0.9 cm × 0.6 cm in size. Several class round lymphatic echogenicity were detected in the level III, VI of left neck with ill-defined margin and unclear cortical medullary margin, one of which were 1.2 cm × 0.7 cm and 0.9 cm× 0.6 cm in level III and VI, respectively.

Lymphatic echogenicity of 1.4 cm × 0.8 cm and 1.4 cm × 1.0 cm in left and right supraclavicular fossa were detected with normal shape and clear cortical medullary margin

CDFI: A small amount of blood flow signals could be observed in the aforementioned lymph nodes.

Sonographic indicates:

Lymphatic echogenicity in left neck (atypical lymph nodes in levelss III and VI)

Lymphatic echogenicity in right neck

Lymphatic echogenicity in bilateral supraclavicular fossa

Fig. 5.3 Sonographic report of Case 16

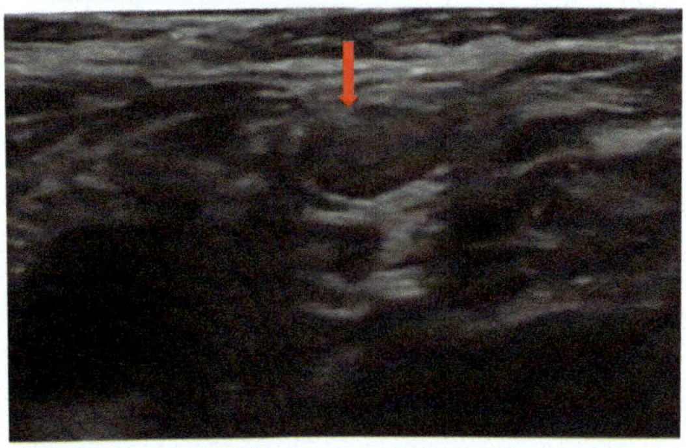

Fig. 5.4 Preoperative ultrasonic reevaluation of Case 16. III. The division of the medullary mass of the lymph nodes in the region is unclear

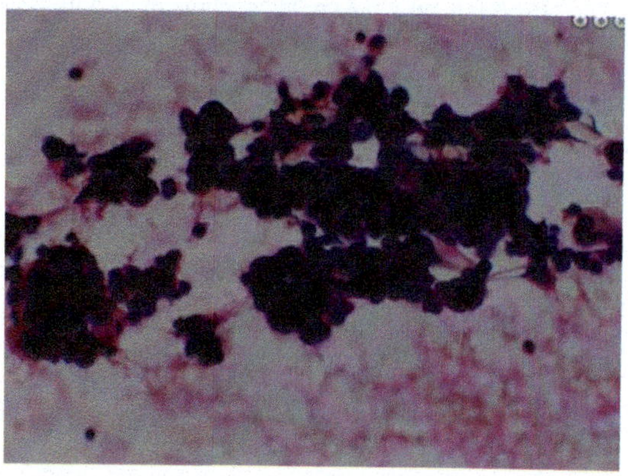

Fig. 5.5 Reports of fine needle aspiration cytology for Case 16. Microscopic visible heterotypic epithelial cells, considering metastatic medullary thyroid carcinoma in conjunction with the medical history. Calcitonin in puncture solution 1799.5 pg/ml ↑(<100 pg/ml)

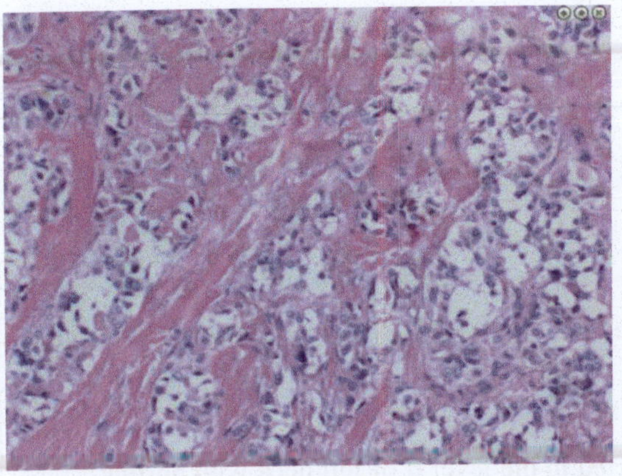

Fig. 5.6 Pathological diagnosis. Metastatic medullary thyroid carcinoma

Case 17

Clinical information: A 35-year-old male patient presented with a hypoechoic nodule in the left lobe (TI-RADS 4b), and a lymph node in level III of left neck with calcification.

Ultrasonic information: Fig. 5.7

Preoperative ultrasound evaluation: Lymph nodes' calcification in level III shown by ultrasound images may consequently be the cross-section of medulla by rotating the probe. Microcalcification has a high possibility of malignancy, but the detection of microcalcification by ultrasound is affected by many factors: first, check whether the ultrasound equipment has

Ultrasonic images:

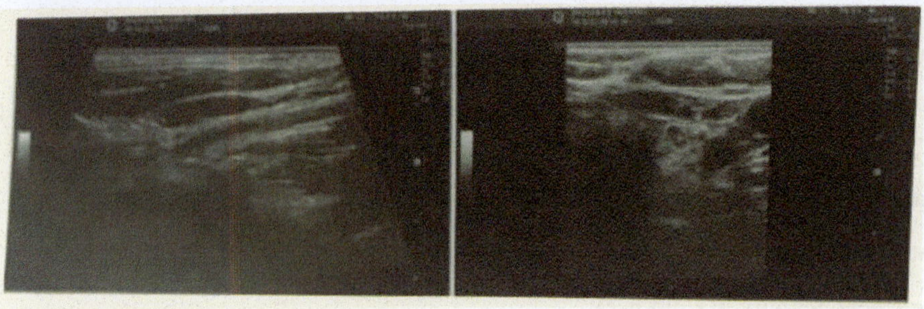

Sonographic findings:

Bilateral neck scan:

Right:

A 0.8 cm × 0.4 cm hypoechoic mass with lymphatic hilum and clear cortex and medulla was detected in level IV of right neck.

Several hypoechoic masses with lymphatic hilum and clear cortex and medulla was detected in level III of right neck one of which was 1.8 cm × 1.7 cm in size.

Left:

A 0.5 cm × 0.3 cm hypoechoic mass with lymphatic hilum and clear cortex and medulla was detected in level VI of left neck.

Several hypoechoic masses with lymphatic hilum and clear cortex and medulla was detected in level IV of left neck, one of which was 0.7 cm × 0.4 cm in size.

Several hypoechoic masses with lymphatic hilum and clear cortex and medulla was detected in level IV of left neck, one of which was 1.4 cm × 0.5 cm in size.

CDFI: Colored blood flow signals are visible in part of the hypoechoic masses.

Sonographic indicates:

Bilateral cervical lymph nodes were detected (nodule in the level III of left neck with calcification)

Fig. 5.7 Sonographic report of Case 17

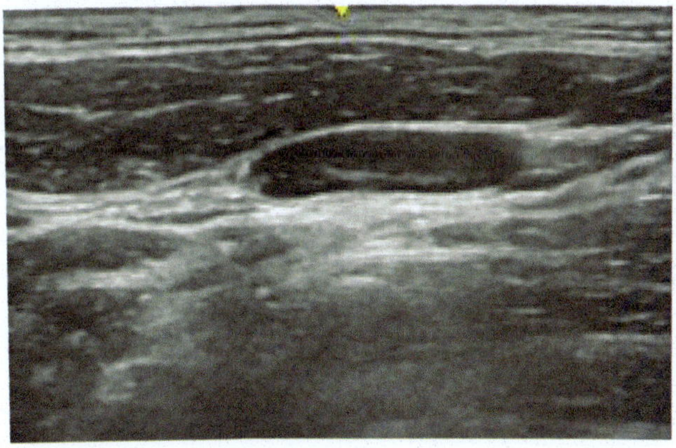

Scan the QR code
to watch the ultrasonic video

Fig. 5.8 Sonographic imaging of Case 17

a good resolution or not. Second, the experience of inspector, correct operating methods, and rigorous scientific attitudes also matter. Third, the size of lesions plays an important role. Lesions or calcifications may be too small to be detected by ultrasound. Fourth, the location of the lesion matters. When the patient is overweight or the location of the lesion is too deep, the microcalcification may be difficult to be observed. Changing for a low-frequency probe may help, but microcalcifications may be neglected. For isolated punctate hyperechogenicity, the probe needs to be turned to exclude the appearance of medulla section (Fig. 5.8).

Pathological diagnosis: Fig. 5.9

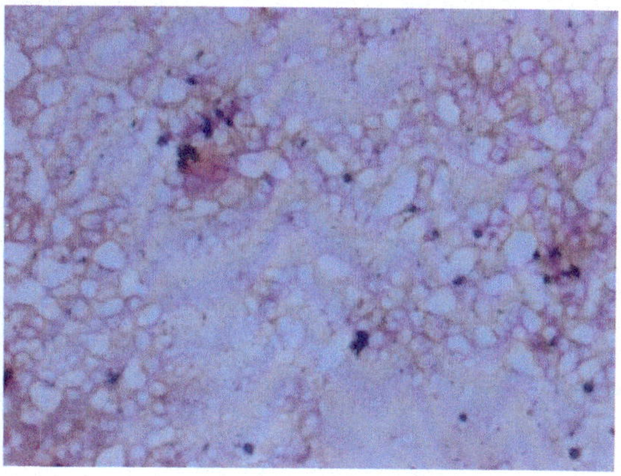

Fig. 5.9 Reports of fine needle aspiration cytology for Case 17. Lymphocytes were visible, but no superior skin cells were observed

Case 18

Clinical information: A 39-year-old female patient was detected with a hypoechoic nodule with punctate calcification in the right lobe, and abnormal shape of lymph node in level III of right neck.

Ultrasonic information: Fig. 5.10

Preoperative ultrasound evaluation: Figs. 5.11, 5.12, and 5.13

Case 19

Clinical information: A 41-year-old male patient presented with cervical mass. T3, T4, and TSH levels were normal. Specialized physical examination: A tough nodule about 2.0*1.5 cm in the left thyroid lobe could be palpated, which moves up and down along with swallowing.

Ultrasonic information: Fig. 5.14

Preoperative ultrasound evaluation: Fig. 5.15

Gross specimen and pathological diagnosis: Figs. 5.16 and 5.17.

Summary: Thyroid ultrasonography plays an important role in the management of surgical strategy. When abnormal lymph node hilum structure, disappearance of dermal medulla, thickening of dermal medulla, and other descriptions were reported, but were not sufficient to diagnose metastasis, clinicians should focus on evaluating these suspected lymph

Ultrasonic images:

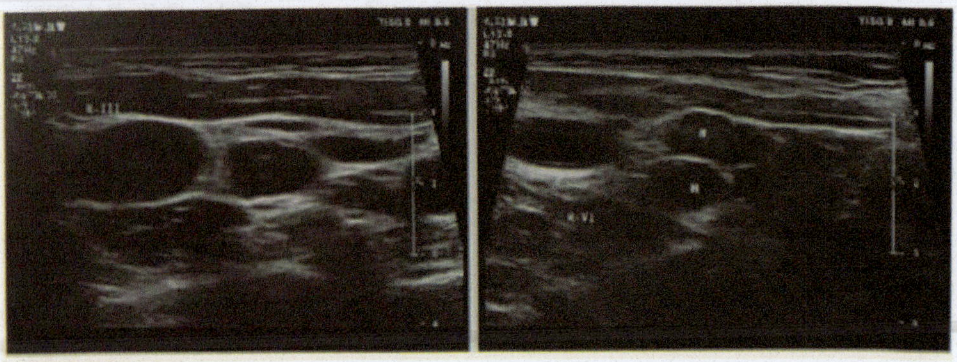

Sonographic findings:

Bilateral neck scan:

Left:

No significant limited echogenicity in the left neck.

Right:

Several hyperechoic masses with dispearred lymphatic hilum in the level II of right neck, one of which was 1.7 cm × 1.2 cm in size.

Several hyperechoic masses with dispearred lymphatic hilum and punctate hyperechogenicity inside in the level III of right neck, one of which was 2.1 cm × 1.1 cm in size.

Several hyperechoic masses with dispearred lymphatic hilum and punctate hyperechogenicity inside in the level IV of right neck, one of which was 1.7 cm × 0.7 cm in size.

Several hyperechoic masses with dispearred lymphatic hilum in the level IV of right neck, one of which was 1.3 cm × 0.7 cm in size.

CDFI: No blood flow signals were observed in the hypoechoic masses.

Sonographic indicates:

Abnormal lymphatic echogenicity in the right neck. (M?)

Fig. 5.10 Sonographic report of Case 18

nodes. It is recommended that ultrasound-guided FNAB cytology or the thyroglobulin (Tg) levels of rinse solution, measured for suspected malignant lymph nodes between 8 mm and 10 mm may help. It is difficult to evaluate the cytology of lymph nodes with most cystic changes. When the results of cytology are inconsistent with the sonographic findings, the level of rinse solution Tg could be regarded as a diagnostic basis.

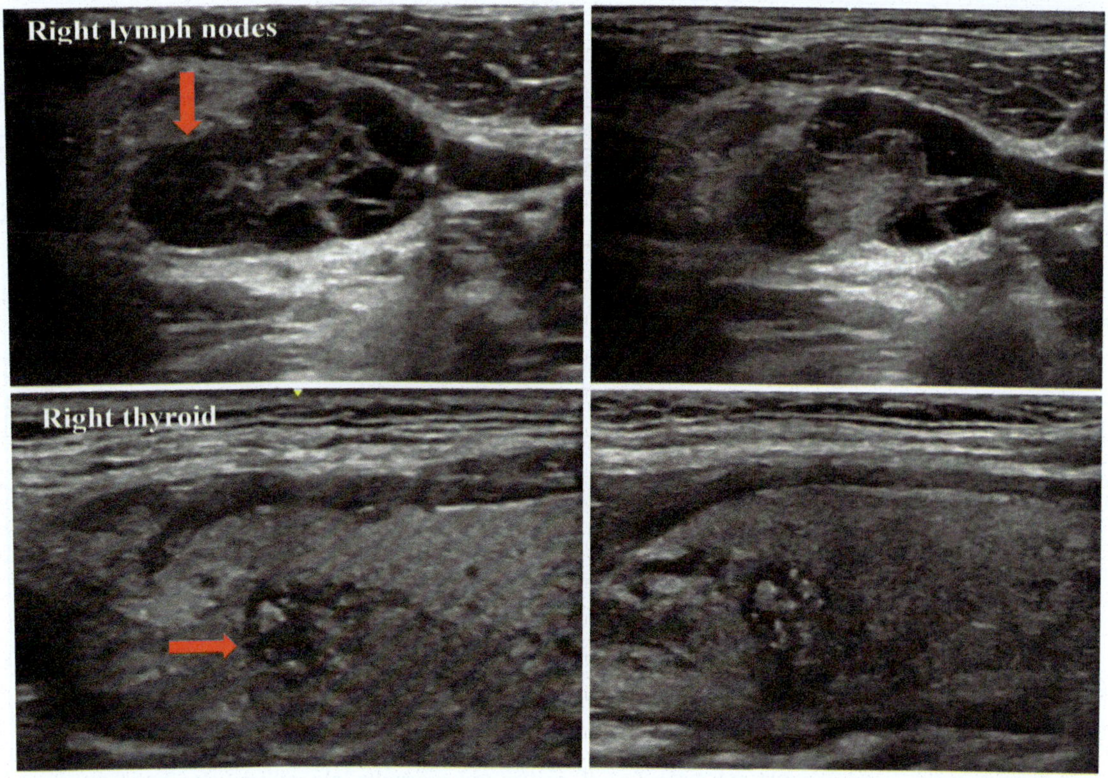

Fig. 5.11 Preoperative ultrasonic reevaluation of Case 18. III. The division of the medullary mass of the lymph nodes in the region is unclear

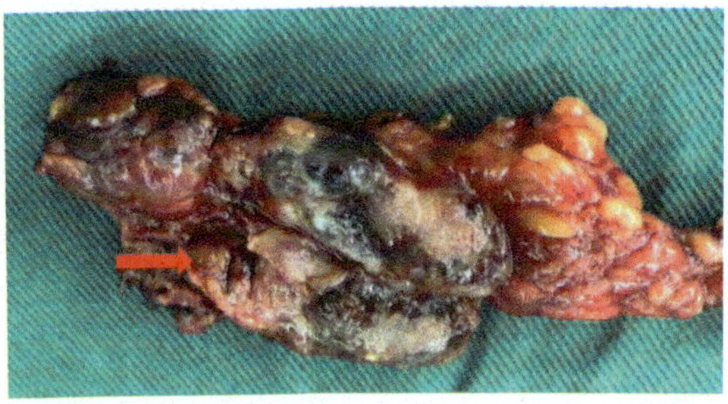

Fig. 5.12 Gross specimen of Case 18. Lymph node specimens are grayish-yellow, grayish-brown with black tissue (nanocarbon)

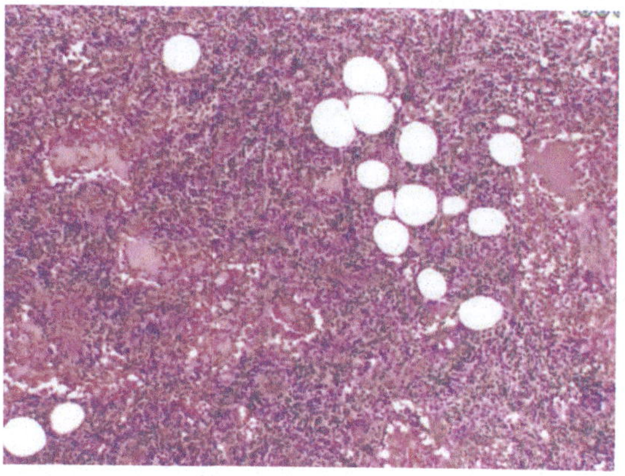

Fig. 5.13 Pathological diagnosis of Case 18. Metastases of papillary thyroid cancer

Sonographic findings:

Scan bilateral neck, axilla, and supraclavicle

Several hypoechoic masses with lymphatic hilum and clear cortex and medulla was detected in level II of bilateral neck, one of which were 1.2 cm × 0.5 cm in the left and 1.8 cm × 0.8 cm in the right.

Two hyperechoic masses with punctate hyperechogenicity inside in the level III of right neck, the size of which were 0.7 cm × 0.3 cm, 1.1 cm × 0.3 cm.

A 1.3 cm × 0.4 cm hyperechoic mass with with lymphatic hilum and clear cortex and medulla in the level IV of left neck.

Several hypoechoic masses with lymphatic hilum and clear cortex and medulla was detected in bilateral axilla, one of which were 1.6 cm × 0.6 cm in the left and 1.6 cm × 0.6 cm in the right.

Several hypoechoic masses with uneven echogenicity inside was detected in bilateral supraclavicle, one of which were 0.7 cm × 0.5 cm in the left and 1.1 cm × 0.3 cm in the right.

CDFI: No blood flow signals were observed in the hypoechoic masses.

Sonographic indicates:

Lymph nodes in the level III of right neck with calcification plaques

Lymph nodes in the level II of bilateral neck, axilla, and supraclavicle without abnormal shape

Fig. 5.14 Sonographic report of Case 19

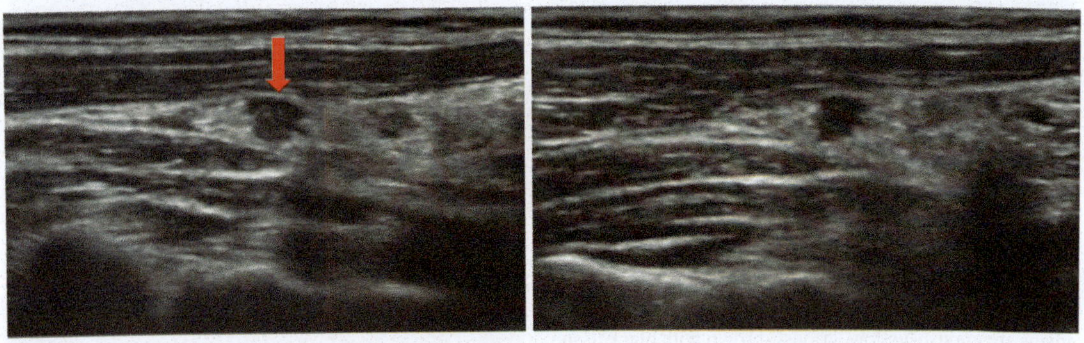

Fig. 5.15 Preoperative ultrasonic reevaluation of Case 19. A 0.7 cm × 0.3 cm lymph node in level III of right neck with abnormal shape and scattered hyperechogenicity inside

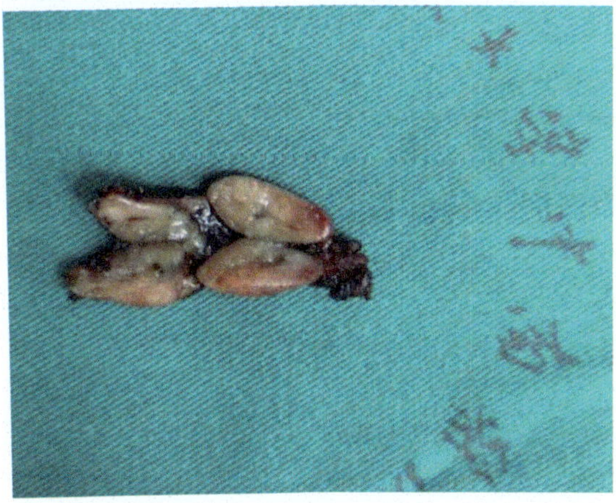

Fig. 5.16 Gross specimen of Case 19

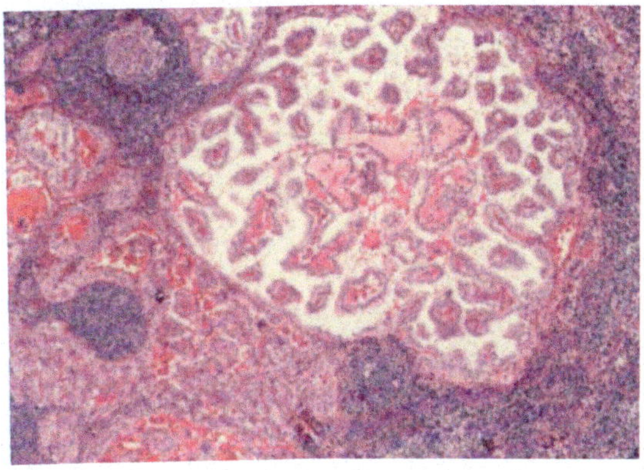

Fig. 5.17 Pathological diagnosis of Case 19. Metastases of papillary thyroid cancer

Further Readings

Li J. Ultrasonic feature analysis of cervical metastatic lymph nodes in thyroid carcinoma. J Hebei Med Univ. 2016;37(6):684–6.

Meng J, Yang G, Wen B, et al. Ultrasonographic differentiation of calcification between cervical tuberculous lymphadenitis and cervical lymph nodes metastasis of papillary thyroid carcinoma. Chin J Ultrasound Med. 2015;31(6):487–9.

Sophie L, Elizabeth G, Mathieu R, et al. Ultrasound criteria of malignancy for cervical lymph nodes in patients followed up for differentiated thyroid cancer. J Clin Endocrinol Metab. 2007;92(9):3590.

Steinkamp HJ, Cornehl M, Hosten N, et al. Cervical lymphadenopathy: ratio of long- to short-axis diameter as a predictor of malignancy. Br J Radiol. 1995;68(3):266–70.

6 Hypoechoic or Hyperechoic Nodules in Parathyroid Glands

6.1 Clinical Overview

Hyperparathyroidism (HPT) refers to parathyroid hormone (PTH) hypersecretion of parathyroid hormone (PTH) due to parathyroid hormone itself or secondary lesions, resulting in calcium, phosphorus, and bone metabolism disorders and a series of clinical manifestations of systemic diseases. According to the etiopathogenesis, parathyroidism hyperactivity can be divided into primary, secondary, and tertiary, and heterologous (pseudo).

Primary hyperparathyroidism (PHPT) is caused by hyperthyroid hormone synthesis and hypersecretion due to parathyroid disease itself; secondary hyperparathyroidism is hypocalcemia caused by various causes, stimulating the parathyroid glands, making them hypertrophiedic, and secreting too much PTH; tertiary parathyroidism hyperactivity is based on secondary hyperparathyroidism. Due to the persistent and intense stimulation of the glands, some hyperplasia tissues turn into adenomas, after the spontaneous secretion of excessive PTH; pseudoparathyroid hyperfunction is due to the malignant tumors of certain organs, such as lungs, kidneys, and ovaries, which secrete peptide substances similar to parathyroid hormones, causing increased blood calcium.

Secondary hyperparathyroidism (SHPT) caused by chronic kidney disease is most common. SHPT is a group of clinical syndromes in which chronic kidney disease occurs hyporenal function, due to decreased active vitamin D synthesis, high blood phosphorus, low blood calcium, and other factors that stimulate the parathyroid glands to increase hypertrophy and secrete excessive parathyroid hormone, causing calcium, phosphorus and bone metabolism disorders, and cardiovascular, neuromuscular, skin, and other multisystem damage.

At present, surgery is its main treatment method, and preoperative detection and accurate localization of lesions are the keys to successful surgery.

6.2 Pathological Type

(1) Adenomas: Mostly a single gland is affected, and seldom have two or more adenomas.

(2) Hyperplasia: Generally four glands are hypertrophied or only one gland is enlarged, mainly cell or water-like transparent cell hyperplasia, there is interstitial fat, the amount of intra-

Supplementary Information The online version contains supplementary material available at https://doi.org/10.1007/978-981-19-8873-8_6.

G. Wu et al., *Pitfalls in Ultrasound of Thyroid Nodules*,
https://doi.org/10.1007/978-981-19-8873-8_6

cellular matrix increases, the shape is different from normal parathyroid tissue, often preserve the lobular structure, but there is no publicly recognized standard for distinguishing adenoma and proliferative morphology.

(3) Adenocarcinoma: Rare, the general tumor body is larger than the adenoma, the growth is slower, the neck examination can often be retracted, it can be regrown after resection, the nucleus is deeply stained, there is nuclear division, there is infiltration of the envelope and blood vessels, local lymph nodes and distant metastasis, metastasis is most commonly seen in the lungs, followed by liver and bone, 3–10% of patients are multiple endocrine adenomas.

6.3 Sonographic Findings

Normal parathyroid glands vary greatly in size, weight, and position, ranging from 4 to 5 mm in diameter and weighing 20–40 mg. Similar to or slightly lower than the thyroid echo, so the parathyroid ultrasound performance has a certain controversy, Wang et al. carried out anatomical measurements and observations of 645 normal human parathyroid glands, the maximum volume was 8 mm× 2 mm× 1 mm, the average was 5 mm× 3 mm× 1 mm, so most authors consider that normal parathyroid ultrasound is difficult to show, only Simeone reported that the normal parathyroid glands were shown with high-resolution ultrasound. Some scholars have shown that normal parathyroid glands are mostly characterized by high echoes. With the development of ultrasound instruments and the advancement of technology, the localization of normal parathyroid glands is completely possible. The enlarged parathyroid glands have different echographic imaging features from surrounding tissues and are therefore easily recognizable. The parathyroid glands are mainly composed of a large number of master cells, a small number of eosinophils and a matrix, the main cells are arranged tightly densely, the cytoplasm is rich in fat particles, and the matrix also contains adipose tissue, so ultrasound is uniformly enhanced echo. When the glands undergo disease changes, such as hyperplasia, adenoma formation, fat droplets in the cytoplasm of the main cell, and fat cells in the interstitium are significantly reduced. The amount of fat content, the richness of the capillary network, and the synthetic secretion status of parathyroid hormone may lead to the diversification of its echo. On ultrasound images, correspondingly changed from strong echo to low echo, and low-echo nodules are the main audiovisual manifestations of parathyroid hyperplasia and adenoma.

The primary parathyroid sonogram is a low-echo mass with a clear boundary, with a variety of forms, mainly oval, round or long, larger adenomas can be lobed or irregular, mostly have a complete envelope, the internal echo is uniform, the peripheral and internal visible and rich arteriovenous blood flow signals, the peripheral blood flow is arc-shaped or circular, and there is a high echo separation band between it and the thyroid gland, which is characteristic of ultrasound diagnosis of parathyroid adenoma (PTA). As the PTA increases in size, especially when the mass is >3 cm in diameter, cystic changes tend to occur, and the glands appear to be echoless due to vascular congestion and rupture ultrasound. Studies have reported that the maximum diameter of 21 PTA with liquefaction is (34.82 ± 7.93) mm, which is significantly greater than the maximum diameter of (18.23 ± 8.54) mm of 49 PTA without liquefaction, which should be diagnosed with thyroid nodule cystic degeneration. The incidence of PTA ectopicity is 26%, the lesion may be located in the tracheal sulcus, thyroid thymus ligament, and upper thymus thoracic inlet. When PHPT is clinically suspected and ultrasound is in the normal position no lesion is found, the possibility of ectopicity should be considered.

Ultrasound image characteristics of secondary hyperparathyroidism: (1) the parathyroid glands are generally bilaterally enlarged, morphologically variable, mostly oval-shaped, round-like, and larger ones can be lobed; (2) the secondary hyperparathyroid glands are enlarged in volume, mostly showing hypoechogenicity, smooth margin, and no obvious capsule; (3) calcified spots can be seen inside larger glands; (4) unproliferated parathyroid blood flow is rare or undetectable; hypertrophic parathyroid blood flow is generally rich, and the surrounding blood flow around the gland is dominant; and (5) Nodules are more common in inferior thyroid glands, about 70%.

Ultrasound images of primary hyperparathyroidism are: (1) sharp margin, smooth, solid hyperechoic nodules; (2) morphologically variable, usually round and oval hypoechogenicity, CDFI often manifests as rich blood flow sign.

Case 20

Clinical information: A female patient was diagnosed with secondary hyperparathyroidism for five years and received regular dialysis for eight years with bone pain, leg numbness, itchy skin, and xerostomia. Preoperative value: PTH 1581.00 pg/mL ↑(14.5–87.5 pg/mL); calcium (Ca^{2+}) 2.96 mmol/L ↑(2.11–2.52 mmol/L); phosphorus (P) 1.77 mmol/L ↑ (0.85–1.51 mmol/L).

Ultrasonic information: Bilateral enlarged parathyroid glands with oval shape, hypoechogenicity, and calcification foci inside were detected (Figs. 6.1, 6.2, 6.3, and 6.4).

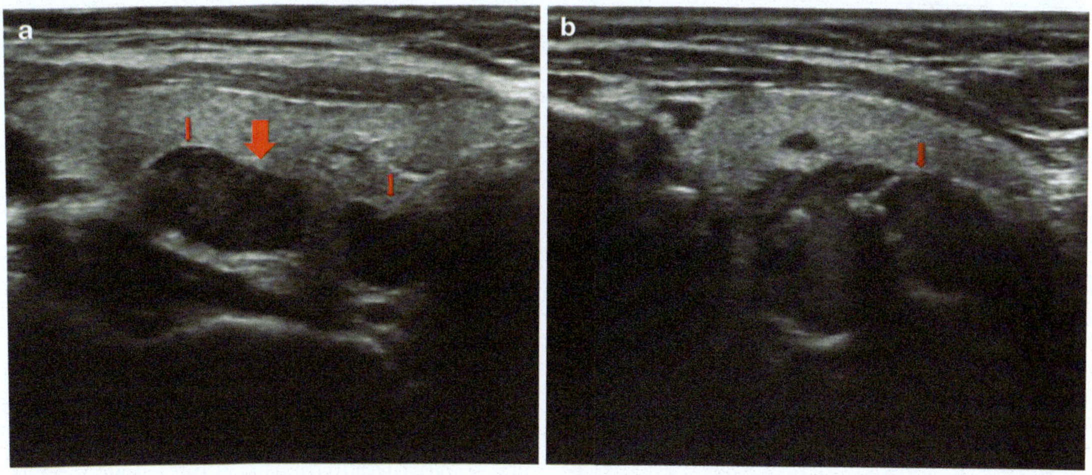

Fig. 6.1 Sonographic report of Case 20 (1). (**a**) Two hyperechoic masses with clear margins were detected in the right parathyroid region, 1.6 cm × 0.9 cm (upper right), 0.9 cm × 0.7 cm (lower right) in size. (**b**) Two hyperechoic masses with clear margins and hyperechoic foci inside were detected in the left parathyroid region, 2.4 cm × 1.3 cm (upper left), 2.5 cm× 1.4 cm (lower left)

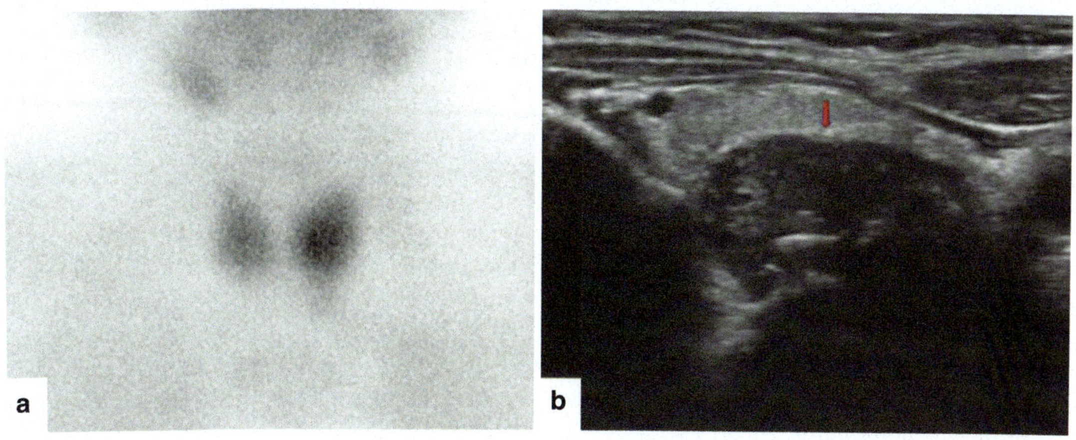

Fig. 6.2 Sonographic report of Case 20 (2). (**a**) Parathyroid imaging: concentration of local radioactivity distribution in the middle and upper left lobe, inferior left lobe, and lower right lobe of the thyroid gland (considered hypertrophic parathyroid tissue, with the highest functional activity of parathyroid tissue in the upper left parathyroid gland); (**b**) Ultrasound shows upper left parathyroid glands 2.5 cm × 1.4 cm in size (lower left) with punctate hyperechogenicity inside

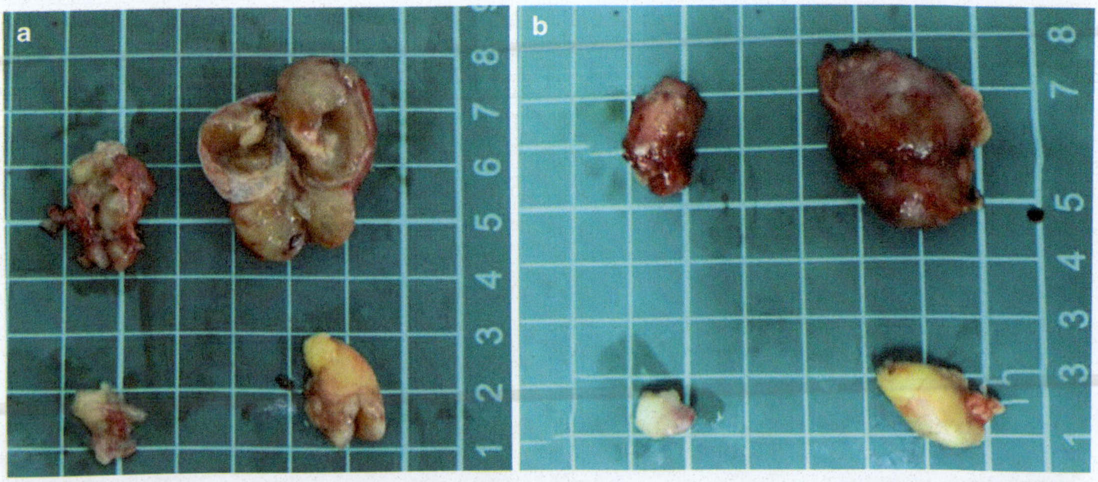

Fig. 6.3 Gross specimen of Case 20. (**a**) Parathyroid specimen with calcified tissue visible in the upper left gland. (**b**) Gross specimen of parathyroid gland

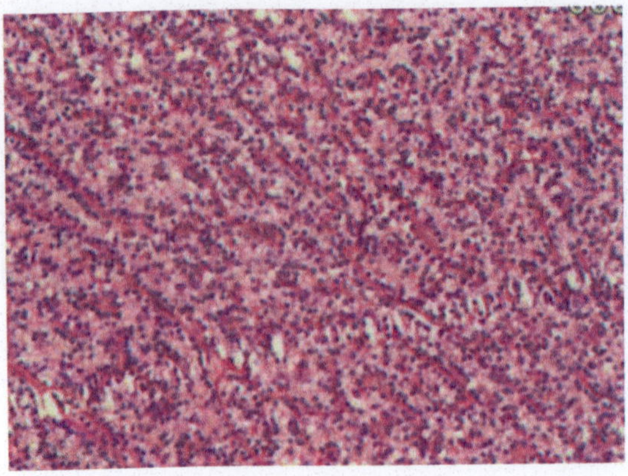

Fig. 6.4 Pathological diagnosis of Case 20. Parathyroid hyperplasia, the gland is mainly composed of master cells, and eosinophils and clear cells can be seen in the nodules of hyperplasia

Case 21

Clinical information: A 34-year-old male patient was diagnosed with chronic renal failure and received regular dialysis for ten years with foot pain for four months. Preoperative value: Ca^{2+} 3.07 mmol/L ↑(2.11–2.52 mmol/L); P: 2.37 mmol/L ↑(0.85–1.51 mmol/L); PTH: 1365.00 pg/mL ↑(14.5–87.5 pg/mL).

Ultrasonic information: Fig. 6.5

Gross specimen and pathological diagnosis: Figs. 6.6 and 6.7

Case 22

Clinical information: A 44-year-old female patient was diagnosed with chronic renal failure and received regular dialysis for 12 years with secondary hyperparathyroidism for four years. Preoperative value: Ca^{2+}: 3.01 mmol/L ↑(2.11–2.52 mmol/L); P: 2.74 mmol/L ↑(0.85–1.51 mmol/L); PTH: 3415.00 pg/mL ↑(14.5–87.5 pg/mL).

Ultrasonic information: Figs. 6.8 and 6.9.

Gross specimen and pathological diagnosis: Figs. 6.10 and 6.11.

Case 23

Clinical information: A 44-year-old male patient was diagnosed with chronic renal failure and received regular dialysis for three years with secondary hyperparathyroidism for half a year. Preoperative value: Ca^{2+}: 2.35 mmol/L (2.11–2.52 mmol/L); P: 2.80 mmol/L↑ (0.85–1.51mmol/L); PTH: 875.00 pg/mL ↑ (14.5–87.5 pg/mL).

Ultrasonic information: Figs. 6.12 and 6.13

Gross specimen and pathological diagnosis: Figs. 6.14 and 6.15

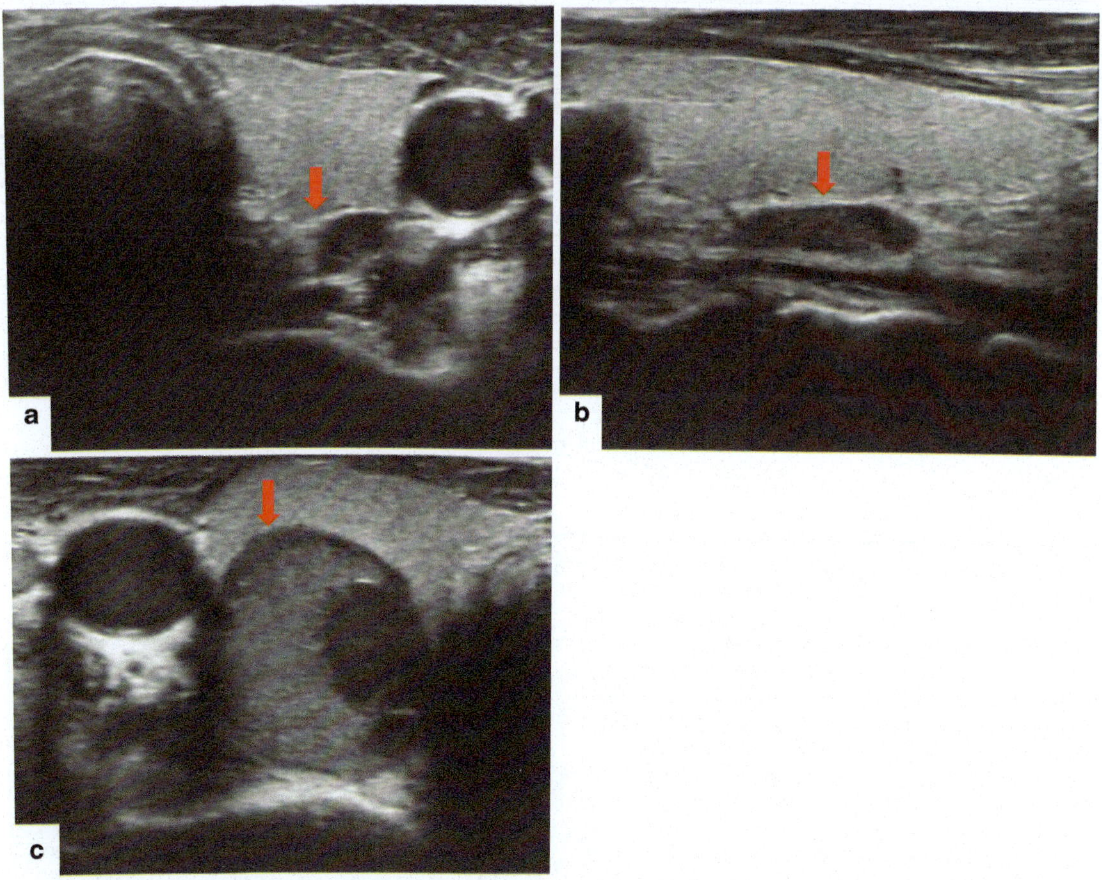

Fig. 6.5 Sonographic report of Case 21. (**a** and **b**) A 1.5 cm × 0.6 cm hyperechoic mass close to the middle and lower left thyroid lobe (red arrow) (**c**) A 3.1 cm × 1.8 cm × 2.1 cm hyperechoic mass with clear margin close to the middle and lower left thyroid lobe (red arrow)

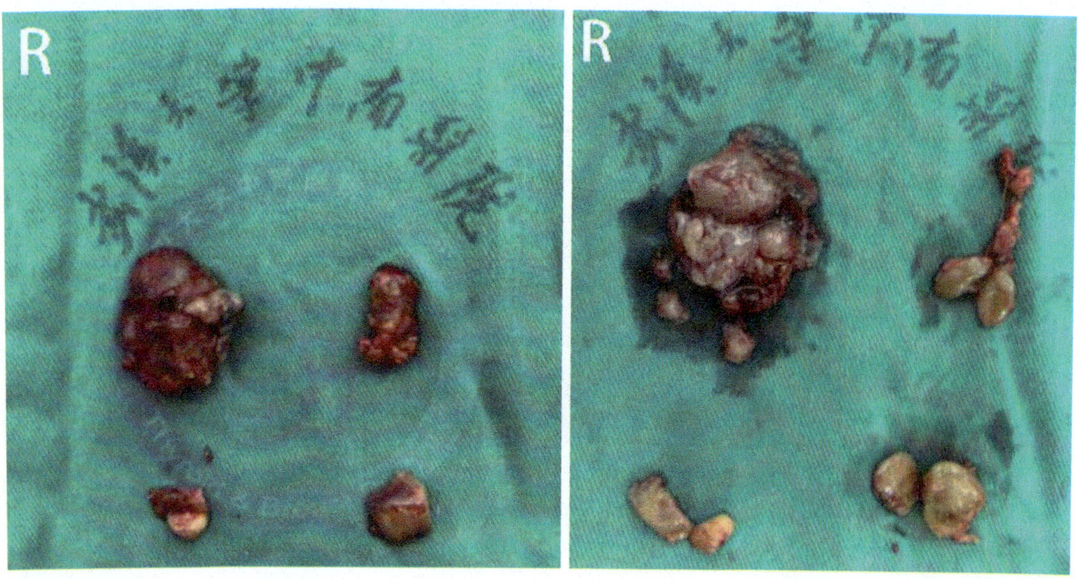

Fig. 6.6 Gross specimen of Case 21

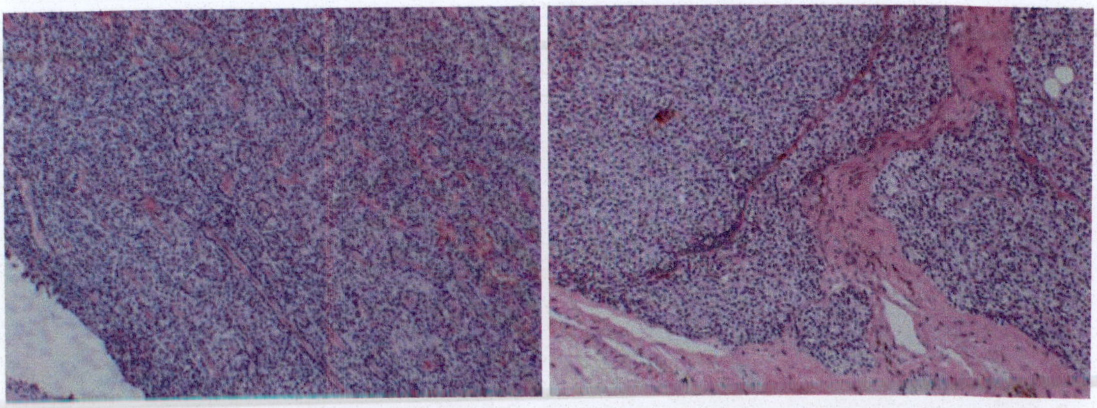

Fig. 6.7 Pathological diagnosis of Case 21: parathyroid hyperplasia

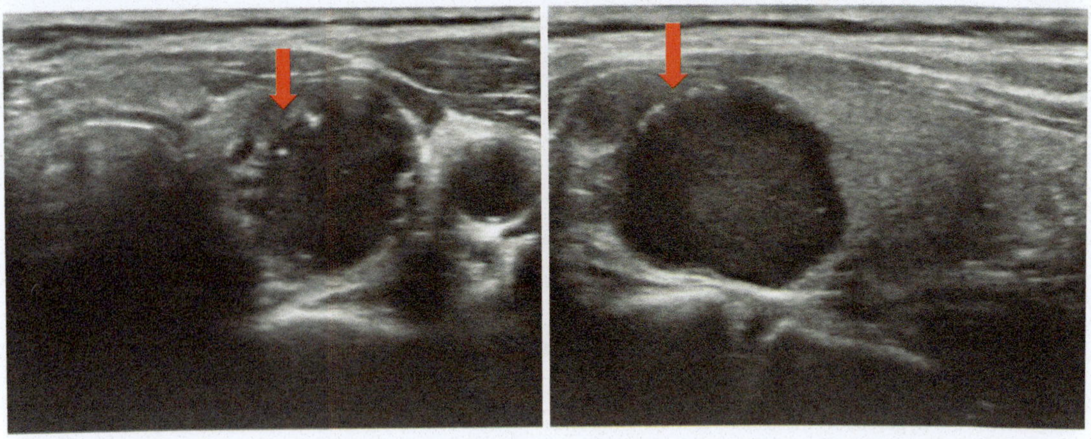

Fig. 6.8 Sonographic report of Case 22 (1). A very low hypoechoic 2.0 cm × 1.8 cm × 1.9 cm in size nodule behind the upper left thyroid lobe

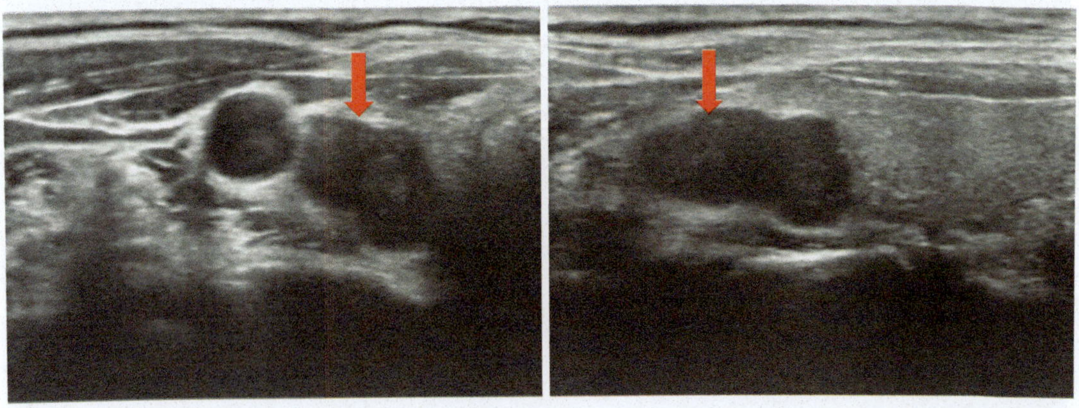

Fig. 6.9 Sonographic report of Case 22 (2). A 1.9 cm × 0.9 cm × 1.1 cm very low hypoechoic mass is visible behind the upper right thyroid lobe, and solid nodules behind the bilateral thyroid lobes (enlarged parathyroid gland?)

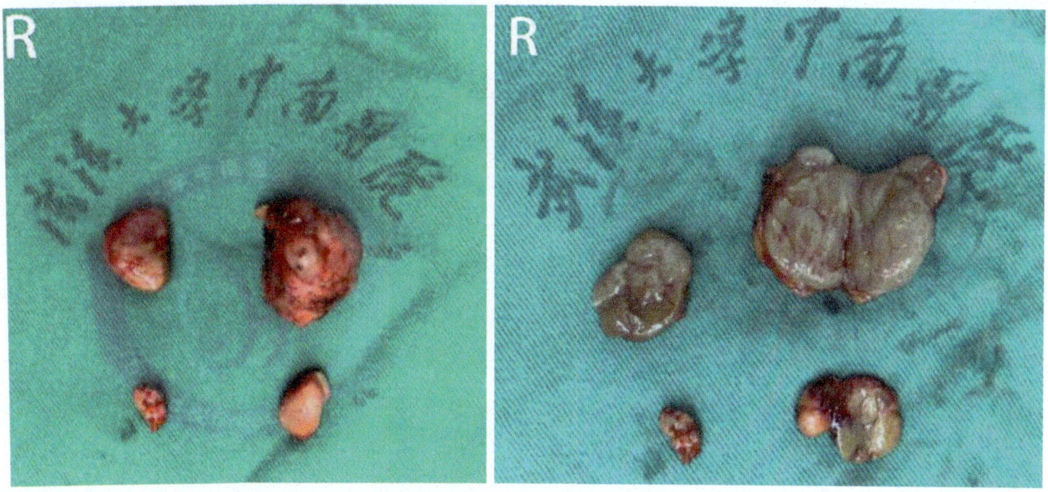

Fig. 6.10 Gross specimen of Case 22. Specimen is gray-brown, tough

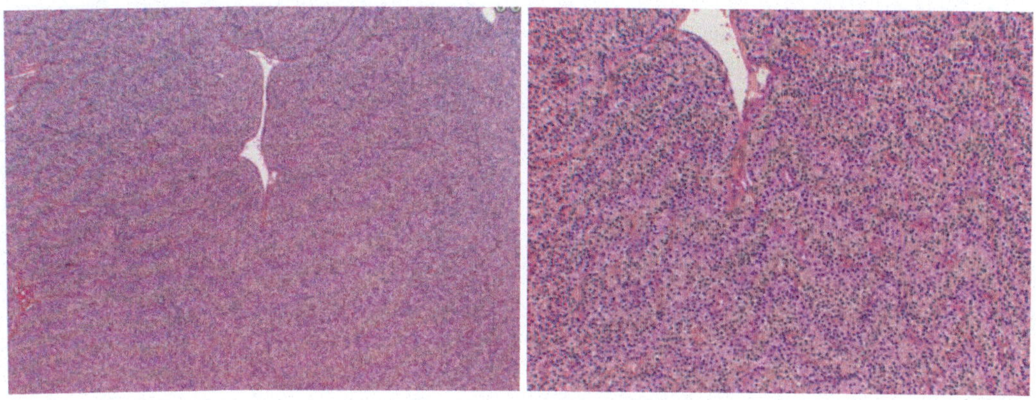

Fig. 6.11 Pathological diagnosis of Case 22: parathyroid hyperplasia

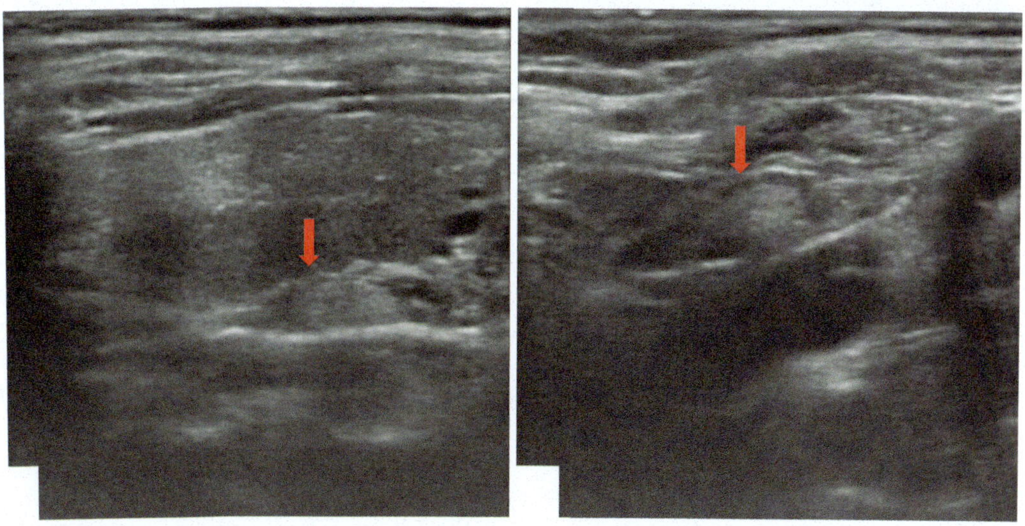

Fig. 6.12 Sonographic report of Case 23. Very high hyperechogenicity in the middle posterior to the bilateral of the thyroid gland and inferior pole of bilateral lobes ((parathyroid glands)?)

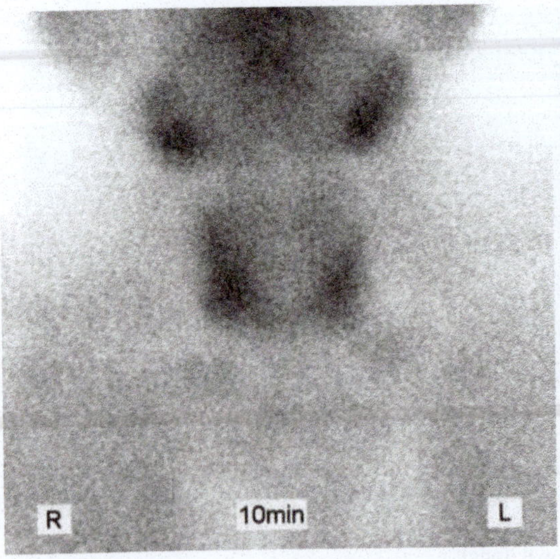

Fig. 6.13 A 0.9 cm × 0.8 cm concentrated shadowing was detected in the middle upper of the left thyroid area. A 0.9 cm × 0.7 cm concentrated shadowing was detected in the middle upper of the right thyroid area. A 1.0 cm × 0.8 cm concentrated shadowing was detected in the middle lower of the left thyroid area. A 1.3 cm × 1.1 cm concentrated shadowing was detected in the middle lower of the right thyroid area

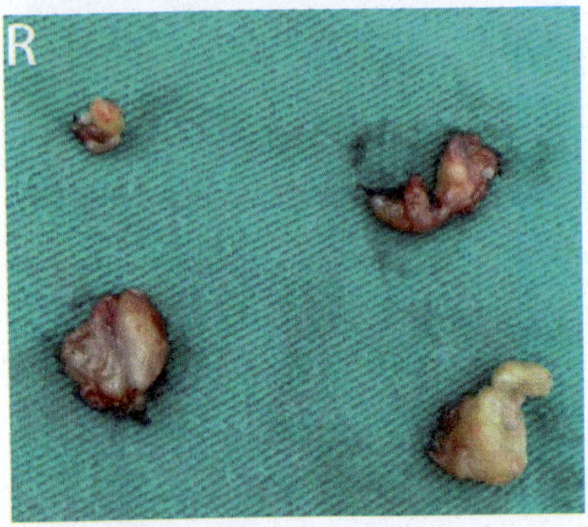

Fig. 6.14 Gross specimen of Case 23

Case 24
Clinical information: A 54-year-old female patient was diagnosed with chronic renal failure

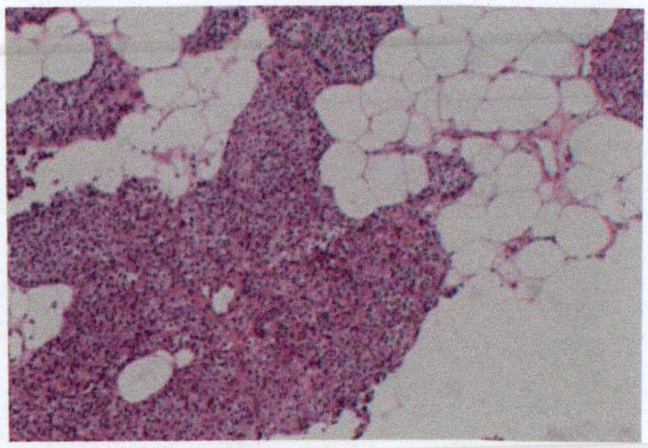

Fig. 6.15 Pathological diagnosis of Case 23. Parathyroid hyperplasia

and received regular dialysis for 13 years with toe and back pain for two years. Preoperative value: Ca^{2+}: 2.09 mmol/L ↓; P: 1.53 mmol/L ↑; PTH: 43.50 pg/mL. The first day after surgery: Ca^{2+}: 1.73 mmol/L ↓; P: 1.34 mmol/L; PTH: 16.60 pg/mL.

Ultrasonic information: Figs. 6.16 and 6.17.

Gross specimen and pathological diagnosis: Figs. 6.18 and 6.19.

Case 25
Clinical information: A 49-year-old female patient was detected with thyroid nodule for three days. Preoperative value: Ca^{2+}: 2.65 mmol/L ↑ (2.11–2.52 mmol/L); P: 0.84 mmol/L ↓ (0.85–1.51 mmol/L); PTH: 300 pg/mL ↑ (14.5–87.5 pg/mL).

Ultrasonic information: Fig. 6.20.

Gross specimen and pathological diagnosis: Fig. 6.21.

Case 26
Clinical information: A 60-year-old male patient diagnosed with repeated renal stone for 20 years, receiving multiple lithotripsy treatment, the treatment effect is not good; the patient is due to bilateral kidney stones, right side hydronephrosis with ureteral stones. During urological hospital-

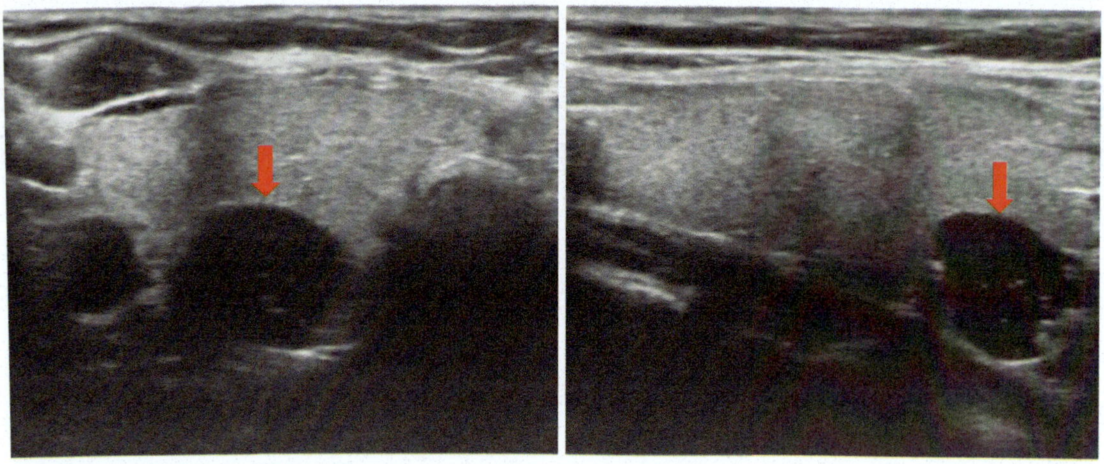

Fig. 6.16 Sonographic report of Case 24 (Left lower parathyroid gland). A very low hypoechogenicity in the left lower thyroid area, 2.5 cm × 1.5 cm in size

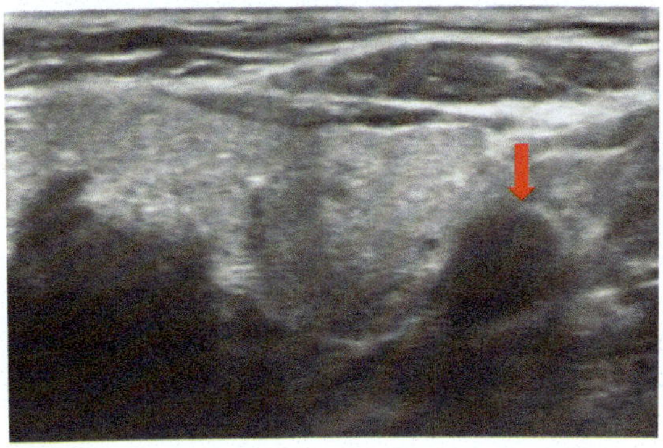

Fig. 6.17 Sonographic report of case 24 Right lower parathyroid gland, 2.5 cm × 1.5 cm

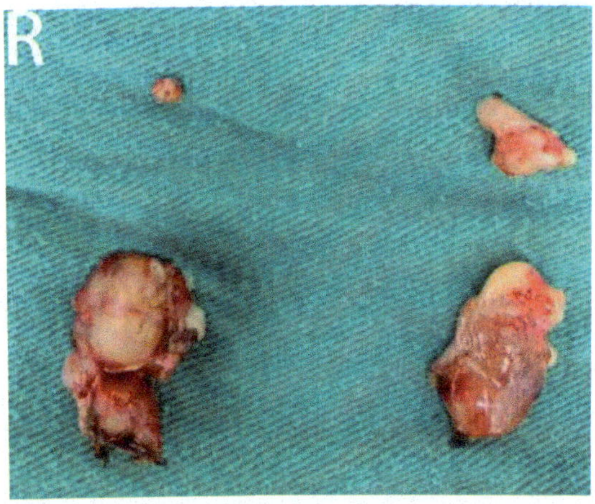

Fig. 6.18 Gross specimen of Case 24

ization, PTH was found increased for one week and turn to the department of thyroid surgery. Bone density-related tests: suggest osteoporosis, thyroid CT scan + enhancement, MIBI imaging of the neck indicate: parathyroid adenoma or hyperplasia of the lower right lobe. Ca^{2+}: 3.32 mmol/L ↑(2.11–2.52 mmol/L); P: 0.51 mmol/L ↓(0.85–1.51 mmol/L); PTH: 292.00 pg/mL ↑(14.5–87.5 pg/mL).

Ultrasonic information: A oval 4.6 cm× 1.7 cm× 1.2 cm hypoechoic mass with clear margin and peripheral punctate blood supply in the lateral left lobe was detected (Figs. 6.20 and 6.22).

Gross specimen and pathological diagnosis: Figs. 6.23 and 6.24.

Case 27

Clinical information: A 63-year-old female patient presented with thyroid nodule without clinical symptom. T3, T4, and TSH levels were normal. Specialized physical examination: A tough nodule about 2.0 cm × 1.0 cm in the left thyroid lobe could be palpated, which moves up and down along with swallowing. PTH: 44.9 pg/mL (14.5–87.5 pg/mL); Ca^{2+}: 2.42 mmol/L (2.11–2.52 mmol/L); P: 1.2 mmol/L (0.85–1.51 mmol/L).

Ultrasonic evaluation: Ultrasound suspects a posterior hypoechoic mass (parathyroid adenoma?) in the middle of the dorsal left lobe (Fig. 6.25).

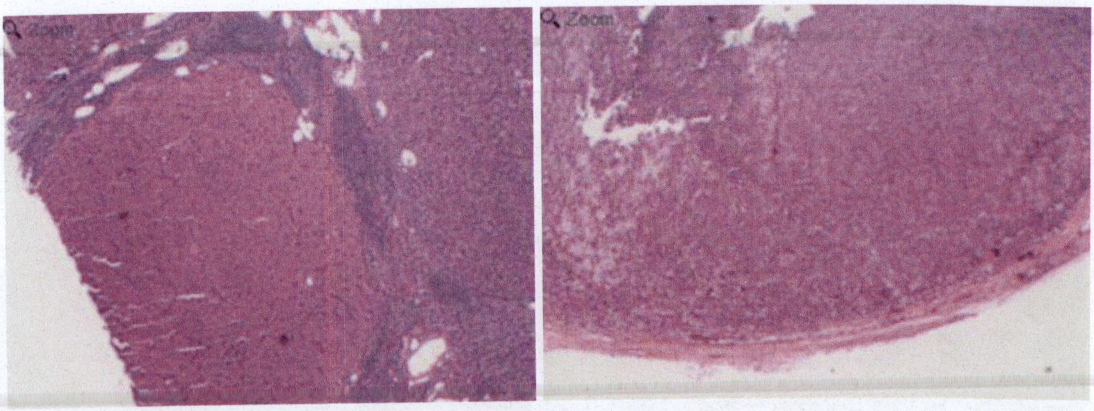

Fig. 6.19 Pathological diagnosis of Case 24: Parathyroid nodular hyperplasia

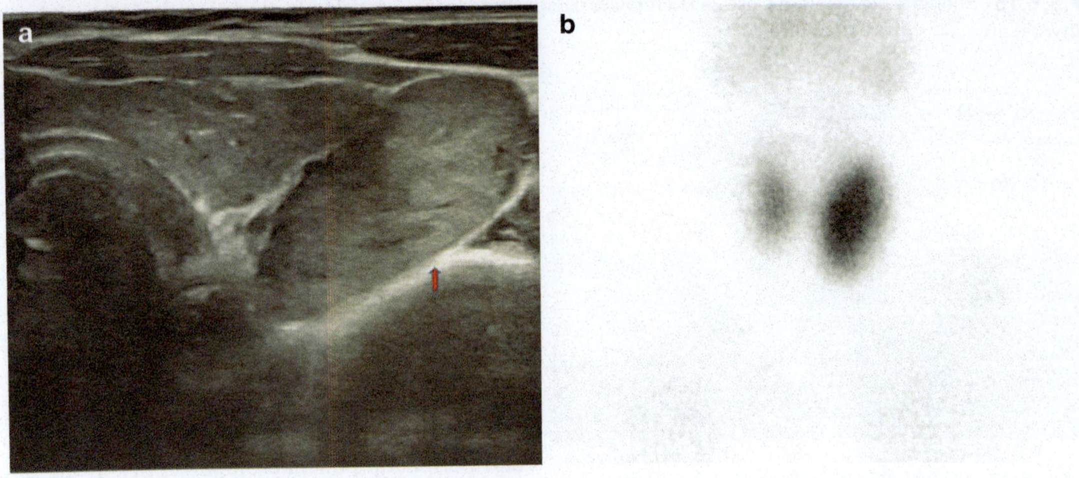

Fig. 6.20 Sonographic report of Case 25. (**a**) A 4.6 cm × 1.7 cm × 1.2 cm isoechoic mass in the lateral of left lobe with clear margin was detected. A distinct linear hyperechogenicity of fibrous fat sacs could be observed between the thyroid gland and the parathyroid glands; (**b**) Abnormally concentrated radiation distribution in the left lobe area of the thyroid gland, considered hyperfunctional parathyroid tissue

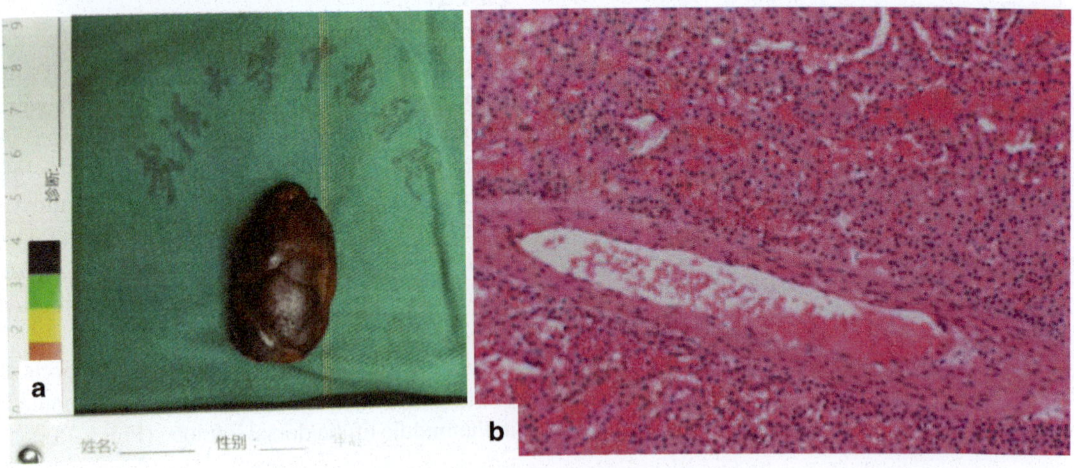

Fig. 6.21 Gross specimen and pathological diagnosis. (**a**) Tissue specimens; (**b**) Diagnosis: parathyroid adenoma

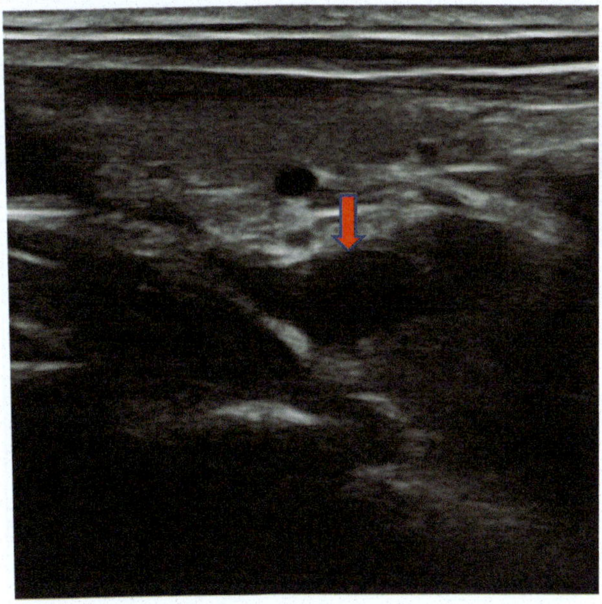

Scan the QR code
to watch the ultrasonic video

Fig. 6.22 Sonographic report of Case 26

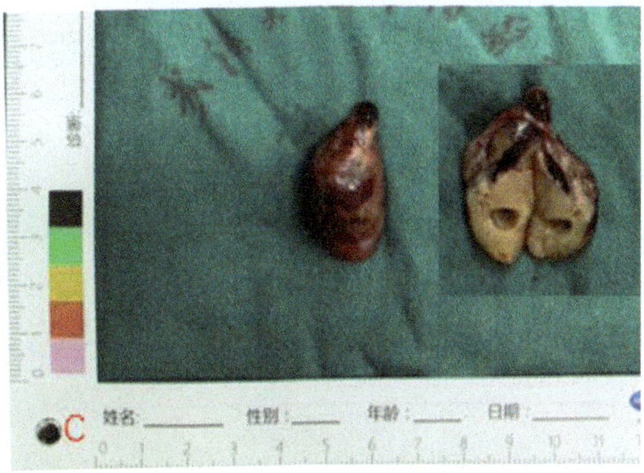

Fig. 6.23 Gross specimen of Case 26. The right upper parathyroid gland is grayish-brown incision

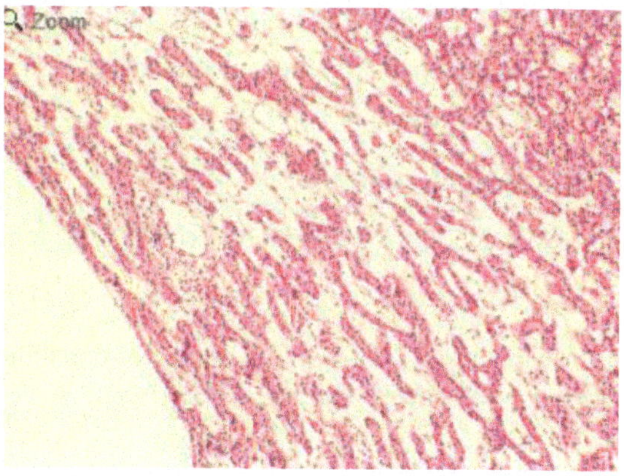

Fig. 6.24 Pathological diagnosis of Case 26. Parathyroid adenoma

Discussion: Misdiagnosis analysis and prevention strategies

Embryos of the parathyroid glands originate in the 3rd and 4th pharyngeal sacs and eventually migrate to the lower neck, therefore the position varies greatly. Usually, the superior parathyroid gland is located in the upper middle one-third of the posterior part of the thyroid lobe, and its position is fixed. The inferior parathyroid gland and thymus jointly originate from the 3rd pharyngeal sac, and together they migrate downward to the neck. Forty-four percent of the inferior parathyroid gland are located less than 1 cm below the thyroid gland, 17% are near the lower thyroid margin, 26% are distributed along the thyroid thymic ligament in the upper part of the thymus, and 2% are located in the thymus gland. The subtopic parathyroid glands may be located in the carotid artery bifurcation, carotid sheath, intrathyroid gland, and posterior pharyngeal wall. Parathyroid echo depends on the fat particles in the cytoplasm of the main cell and the adipose

Ultrasonic images:

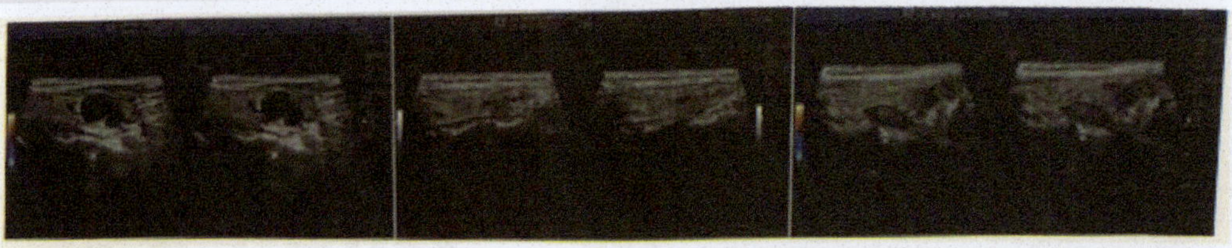

Sonographic findings:

Thyroid scan

Left lobe: 5.0 × 1.7 × 1.4 cm.

Right lobe: 4.5 × 1.2 × 1.0 cm.

Isthmus: anteroposterior diameter is 0.23 cm.

Size and shape were abnormal on thyroid transverse view. The echogenicity of parenchyma is uneven. A mixed echoic 2.1 cm × 1.2 cm nodule with clear margin, anechoic and isoechoic area inside in the inferior of left lobe. A mixed echoic 0.7 cm × 0.3 cm nodule with clear margin, anechoic and isoechoic area inside in the inferior of right lobe. Several anechoic areas with clear margin and hyperechoic foci inside were detected in the right lobe, one of which was 0.5 cm × 0.3 cm.

A hypoechoic1.7 cm × 0.7 cm nodule with clear margin and uneven echogenicity inside in the middle of dorsal left lobe was observed.

CDFI: Colored blood flow signals were visible in the aforementioned nodules.

Sonographic indicates:

Mixed echogenicity in the bilateral thyroid lobes (TI-RADS 3)

Anechoic area in the right lobe (colloid cyst)

A hypoechoic nodule in the middle of dorsal left lobe (parathyroid adenoma?)

Fig. 6.25 Sonographic report of Case 27

tissue in the matrix, due to the small size and position of the parathyroid glands the concealment and anatomical variations bring certain difficulties to ultrasound detection. Secondary parathyroid hyperplasia, due to the presence of a complete envelope and peripheral vascular surroundings, using high-frequency color ultrasound exploration, more than 75% of patients can obtain satisfactory images, and their characteristic ultrasound image performance has become the clinician's preferred method for diagnosing parathyroid hyperplasia and observing the therapeutic effect of secondary hyperparathyroidism.

There are four possible reasons for the difficulty of parathyroid diagnosis: (1) There are dynamic changes in the fat composition of the normal parathyroid gland, and when the content is small, the difference in acoustic impedance with the surrounding structure is low, which is not enough to form a clear boundary; when the gland is diseased, the main cells decrease, the fat particles are also reduced, and the fat content, the richness of the capillary network and the synthetic secretion of parathyroid hormone may lead to the diversification of echogenicity. (2) Ultrasound physicians have limited operation techniques and insufficient awareness of atypical parathyroid glands. (3) Difficulty distinguishing from normal thyroid nodules. Generally, the nails are multiple, unclear boundaries, unequal sizes, and different echo intensities of nodules; ectopic parathyroid glands are single, uniformly hypoechogenicity with clear margins; nails are dominated by few blood flow nodules. (4) Differentiation from lymph nodes. Hyperplasia of the parathyroid gland is mainly oval and irregular, the length and short diameter are not much different; the lymph nodes are flat and round, or flattened, the length is significantly larger than the short diameter; ultrasound images show that there are blood vessels surrounding the parathyroid glands, and see branches into the gland; while there are no blood vessels outside the lymph nodes, only the blood vessels are seen in the lymphatic portal into the node. In the case of the above doubts, the probe can be rotated, and the possibility of parathyroid glands can be ruled out, if the strip long axis section or strip blood flow of the above organ can be displayed.

Further Readings

Li X, Qian H, Li J. Chief physician of endocrinology 1231 questionnaire, vol. 05. Beijing: Military Medical Science Press; 2012. p. 154.

Yao K, Singer FR, Roth SI, Sassoon A, Ye C, Giuliano AE. Weight of normal parathyroid glands in patients with parathyroid adenomas. J Clin Endocrinol Metab. 2004;89:3208–13.

Zhao C, Zhang X. Application progress of ultrasound in diagnosis and treatment of primary hyperparathyroidism. J Clin Ultrasound Med. 2019;021(006):446–8.

Zhang J-Q, Huang B-Z, Mei C-L. Ultrasonography of secondary hyperparathyroidism. Acad J Sec Med Univ. 2002;23(11):1252–4.

7 Analysis of Thyroid Ultrasound Cases

Professor Wu has about 1,000 outpatient visits in one month and performed about 1,000 thyroid surgeries in one year, of which thyroid carcinoma about 800 times. Dr. Wu has accumulated a large number of cases over the years. Here, we categorized the common thyroid ultrasound cases.

7.1 Category 1: TI-RADS 4a or 4b Thyroid Nodules with Obvious Malignant Signs

Case 28: Hypoechoic Nodule

Clinical information: A 4-year-old male patient was detected with left thyroid nodule for 3 years. Specialized physical examination: A tough nodule about 0.5 cm × 0.4 cm in the left thyroid lobe could be palpated, which moves up and down along with swallowing.

Ultrasonic information: Fig. 7.1

Preoperative ultrasound evaluation: Ultrasonic characteristics: Spherical irregular hypoechogenicity with punctate hyperechogenicity inside was observed in the left thyroid lobe (Fig. 7.2).

Gross specimen and pathological diagnosis: Figs. 7.3 and 7.4.

Case 29: Taller than Wide

Clinical information: A 41-year-old male patient was detected with thyroid nodule without clinical symptoms. T3, T4, and TSH levels were normal.

Ultrasonic information: Figs. 7.5 and 7.6

Gross specimen and pathological diagnosis: Figs. 7.7 and 7.8.

Case 30: Taller than Wide

Clinical information: A 52-year-old female patient was detected with right thyroid nodule for one week. T3, T4, and TSH levels were normal.

Ultrasonic information: Fig. 7.9

Preoperative ultrasound evaluation: Fig. 7.10

Gross specimen and pathological diagnosis: Figs. 7.11 and 7.12.

Case 31: Taller than Wide

Clinical information: A 38-year-old male patient was detected with left thyroid nodule for one month. T3, T4, and TSH levels were normal.

Ultrasonic information: Fig. 7.13

Preoperative ultrasound evaluation: Fig. 7.14

Gross specimen and pathological diagnosis: Figs. 7.15 and 7.16.

Supplementary Information The online version contains supplementary material available at https://doi.org/10.1007/978-981-19-8873-8_7.

G. Wu et al., *Pitfalls in Ultrasound of Thyroid Nodules*,
https://doi.org/10.1007/978-981-19-8873-8_7

Ultrasonic images:

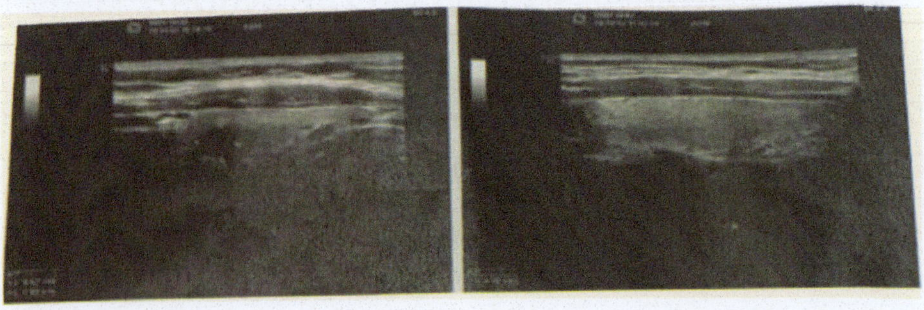

Sonographic findings:

Thyroid scan

Left lobe: 3.9 × 1.3 × 1.3 cm.

Right lobe: 4.1 × 1.2 × 1.4 cm.

Isthmus: anteroposterior diameter is 0.22 cm.

Size and shape were normal on thyroid transverse view. No obvious limited echogenicity was detected in the right lobe. A taller than wide 0.67 cm × 0.69 cm hypoechoic foci with clear margin and irregular shape was observed in the middle upper of left lobe.

CDFI: Colored blood flow signals were not significantly increased in the thyroid.

Sonographic indicates:

Hypoechoic nodule in the left lobe (TI-RADS 4a)

Fig. 7.1 Sonographic report of Case 28

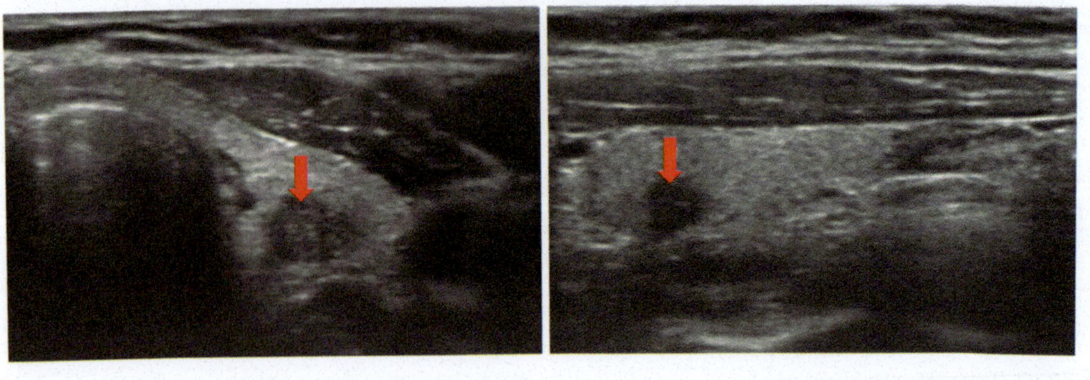

Fig. 7.2 Preoperative ultrasonic reevaluation of Case 28

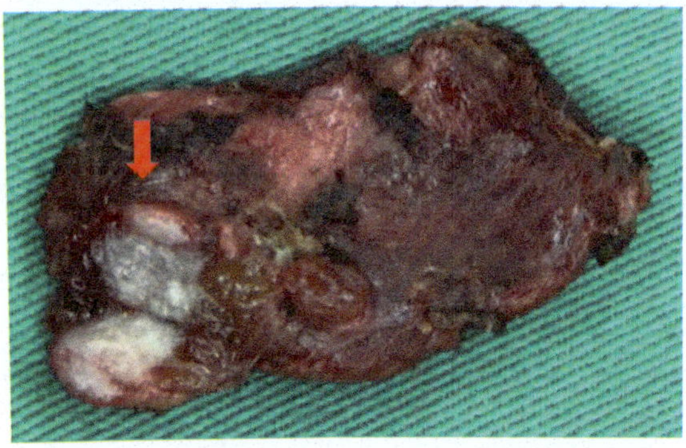

Fig. 7.3 Gross specimen of Case 28. A 0.3-cm grayish-brown nodule

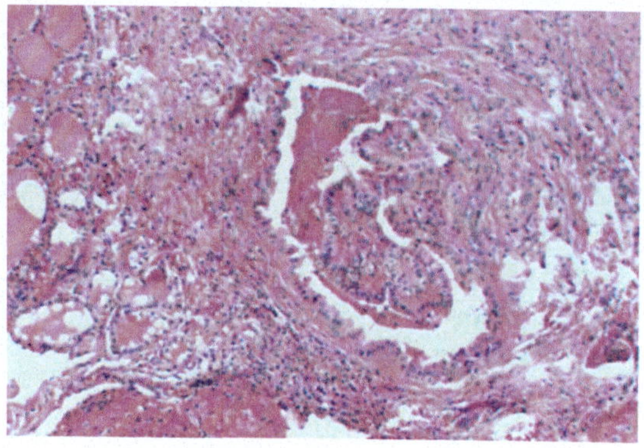

Fig. 7.4 Pathological diagnosis of Case 28. Papillary thyroid microcarcinoma

Ultrasonic images:

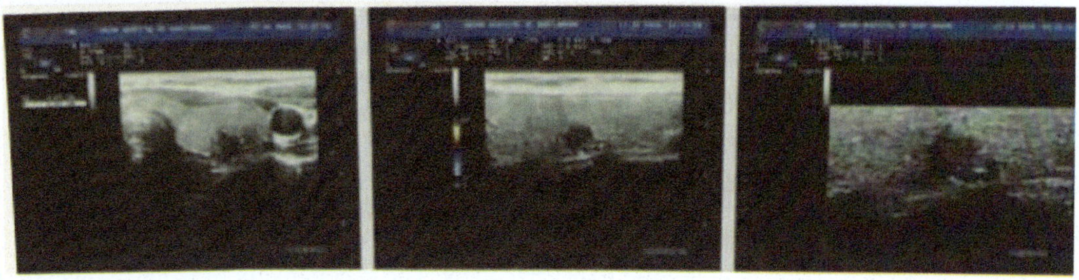

Sonographic findings:

Size and shape were normal on thyroid transverse view. A taller than wide 0.67 cm × 0.69 cm hypoechoic foci with ill-defined margin was observed in the middle dorsal of left lobe.

CDFI: Colored blood flow signals were not significantly increased in the nodule.

Sonographic indicates:

Solid taller than wide nodule in left lobe with ill-defined margin.

Fig. 7.5 Sonographic report of Case 29

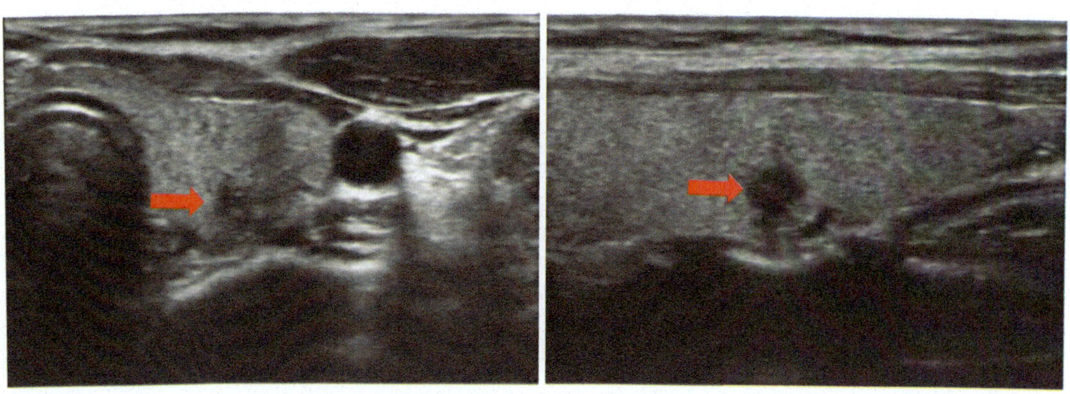

Fig. 7.6 Preoperative ultrasonic reevaluation of Case 29

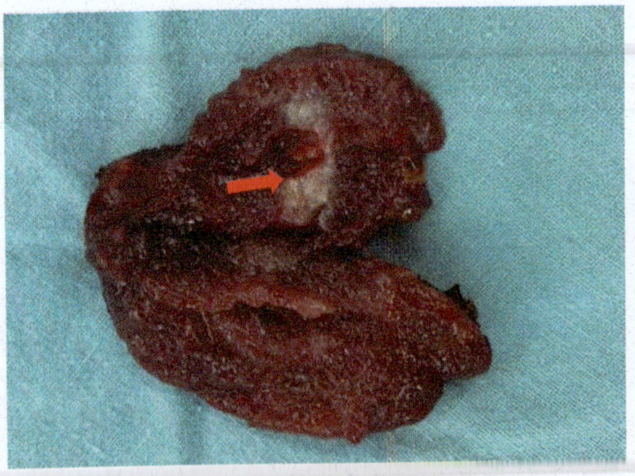

Fig. 7.7 Gross specimen of Case 29. A 0.8-cm gray and white nodules with ill-defined margin with surrounding tissue

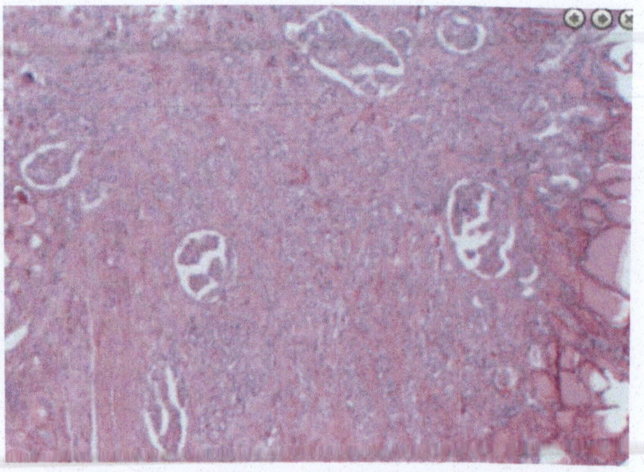

Fig. 7.8 Pathological diagnosis of Case 29. Left papillary thyroid carcinoma, invading fiber adipocyte, does not break through the capsule

Sonographic findings:

Thyroid scan

Left lobe: 5.0 cm × 1.4 cm × 1.3 cm.

Right lobe: 4.7 cm × 1.2 cm × 1.4 cm.

Isthmus: anteroposterior diameter is 0.27 cm.

Size and shape were normal on thyroid transverse view. The echogenicity of parenchyma is sightly low and uneven. A taller than wide 0.63 cm × 0.73 cm hypoechoic foci with ill-defined margin and irregular shape was observed in the superior of right lobe.

CDFI: Colored blood flow signals were not significantly increased in the hypoechoic foci.

Sonographic indicates:

Diffuse lesions of the thyroid gland

Hypoechoic nodule in the right lobe (TI-RADS 4b)

Fig. 7.9 Sonographic report of Case 30

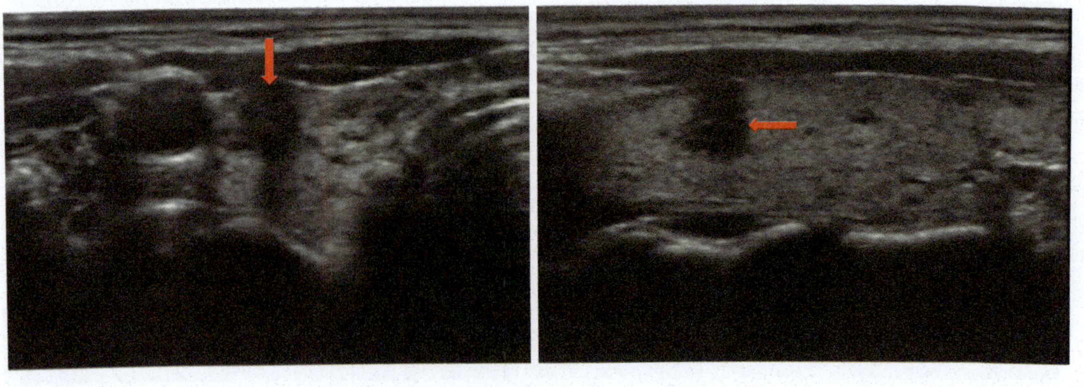

Fig. 7.10 Preoperative ultrasonic reevaluation of Case 30

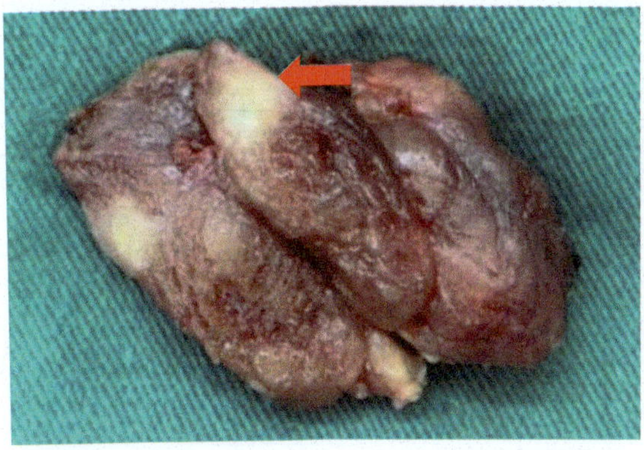

Fig. 7.11 Gross specimen of Case 30. A gray and white nodule was observed

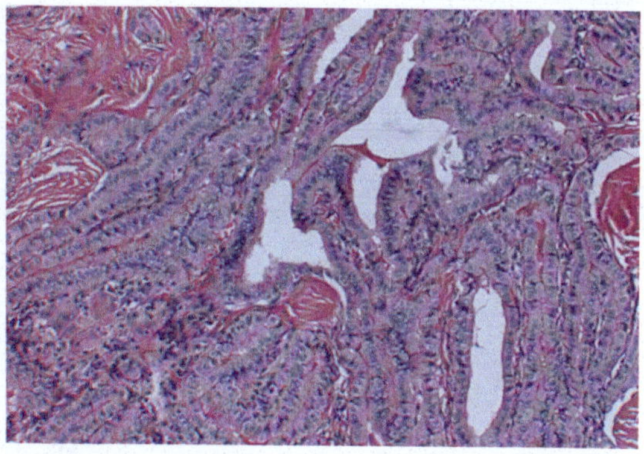

Fig. 7.12 Pathological diagnosis of Case 30. Papillary thyroid carcinoma

Ultrasonic images:

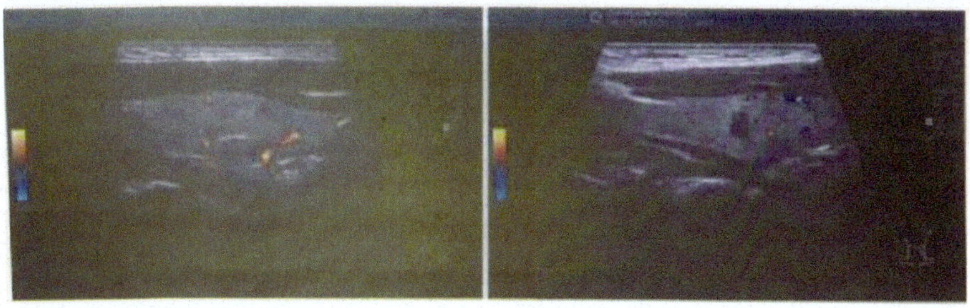

Thyroid scan

Left lobe: 5.3 cm × 1.4 cm × 1.6 cm.

Right lobe: 4.9 cm × 1.3 cm × 1.6 cm.

Isthmus: anteroposterior diameter is 0.31 cm.

Size and shape were normal on thyroid transverse view. The echogenicity of parenchyma and uneven. A taller than wide 0.43 cm × 0.56 cm hypoechoic nodule with ill-defined margin and uneven echogenicity inside was observed in the middle of left lobe.

CDFI: Colored blood flow signals were not significantly increased in the hypoechoic nodule.

Sonographic indicates:

Hypoechoic nodule in the left lobe (TI-RADS 4b)

Fig. 7.13 Sonographic report of Case 31

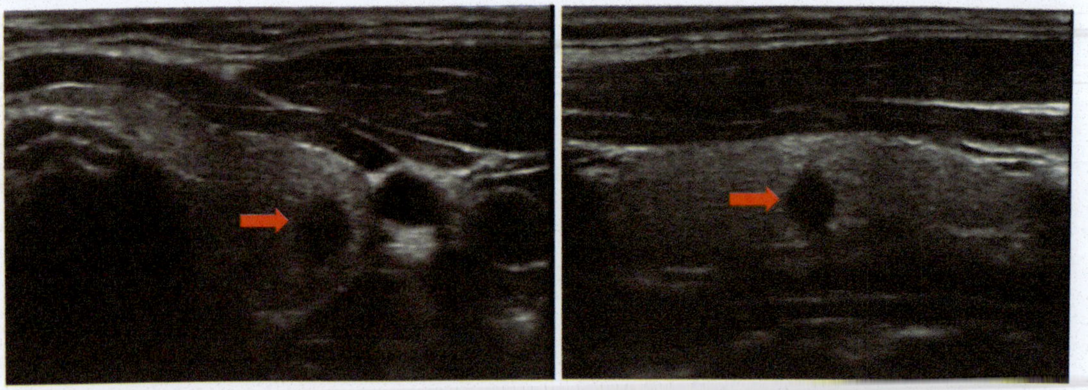

Fig. 7.14 Preoperative ultrasonic reevaluation of Case 31: A taller than wide hypoechoic nodule

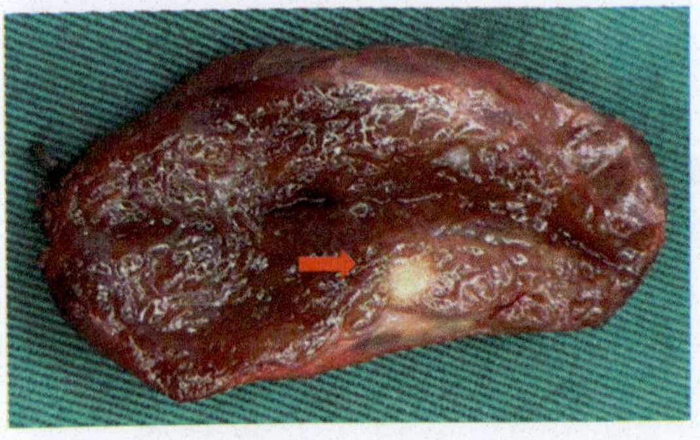

Fig. 7.15 Gross specimen of Case 31. A 0.4-cm gray and white nodule

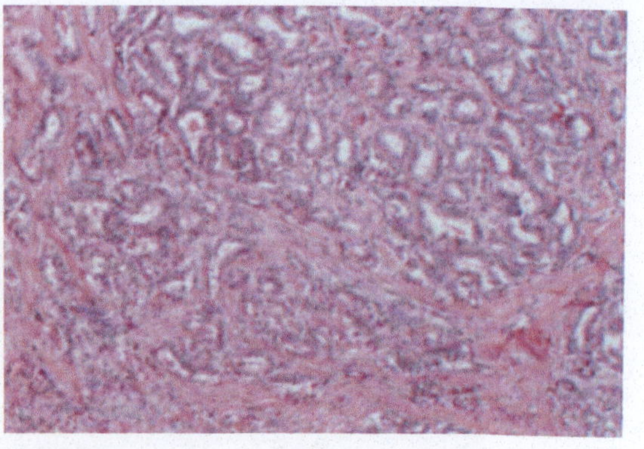

Fig. 7.16 Pathological diagnosis of Case 31: Papillary thyroid carcinoma

Case 32: Taller than Wide

Clinical information: A 52-year-old female patient was detected with thyroid nodule for one week without clinical symptoms. T3, T4, and TSH levels were normal.

Ultrasonic information: Fig. 7.17

Preoperative ultrasound evaluation: Fig. 7.18

Gross specimen and pathological diagnosis: Figs. 7.19, 7.20, and 7.21.

Case 33: Taller than Wide, Hypoechogenicity, and Calcification

Clinical information: A 38-year-old female patient was detected with right thyroid nodule for two years. T3, T4, and TSH levels were normal. FT3: 5.04 pmol/L (3.21–6.5 pmol/L), FT4 20.33 pmol/L (10.22–21.88 pmol/L), TSH 0.859 μU/mL (0.3–4.6 μU/mL), Anti-Tg 577 U/mL ↑(0–72 U/mL), A-TPO 6 U/mL (0–16 U/mL).

Ultrasonic information: Fig. 7.21

Gross specimen and pathological diagnosis: Figs. 7.22 and 7.23.

Case 34: Hypoechogenicity and Tend to Be Spherical

Clinical information: A 53-year-old female patient was detected with right thyroid nodule for half a year. T3, T4, and TSH levels were normal.

Ultrasonic images:

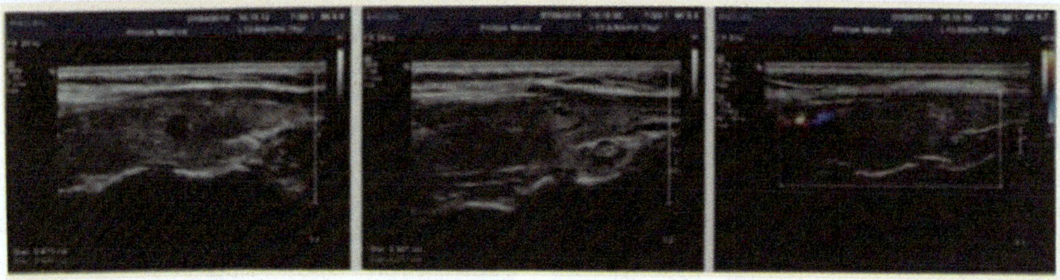

Sonographic findings:

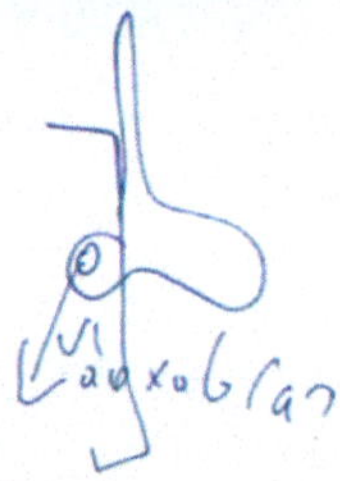

Thyroid scan

Left lobe: 4.5cm× 1.5cm× 1.4cm.

Right lobe: 4.5cm× 1.5cm× 1.4cm.

Isthmus: anteroposterior diameter is 0.2 cm.

The echogenicity of parenchyma was uniform. A taller than wide 0.4 cm × 0.6 cm hypoechoic foci with ill-defined margin and irregular shape was observed in the of right lobe. And an anechoic nodule was observed in the right lobe.

CDFI: No blood flow signals were observed in the hypoechoic foci.

Sonographic indicates:

吴高松

Hypoechoic foci in the right lobe (TI-RADS 4b)

Cyst in the right lobe (TI-RADS 2)

Fig. 7.17 Sonographic report of Case 32

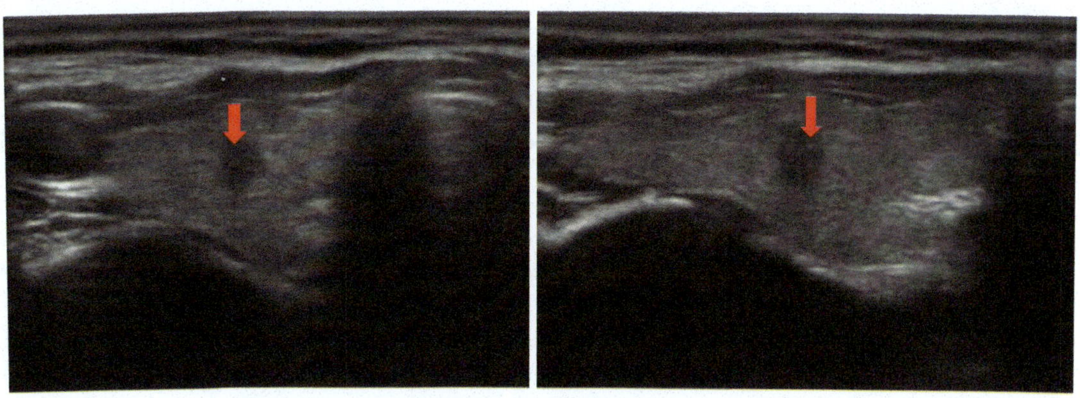

Fig. 7.18 Preoperative ultrasonic reevaluation of Case 32. A taller than wide hypoechoic nodule in the right lobe

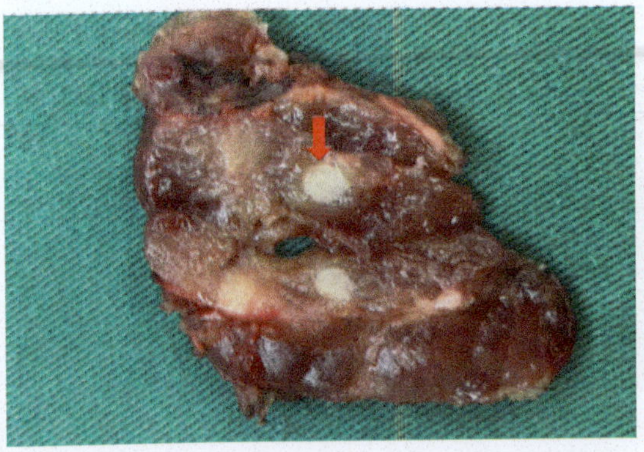

Fig. 7.19 Gross specimen of Case 32. A 0.5-cm gray and white nodule with clear margin

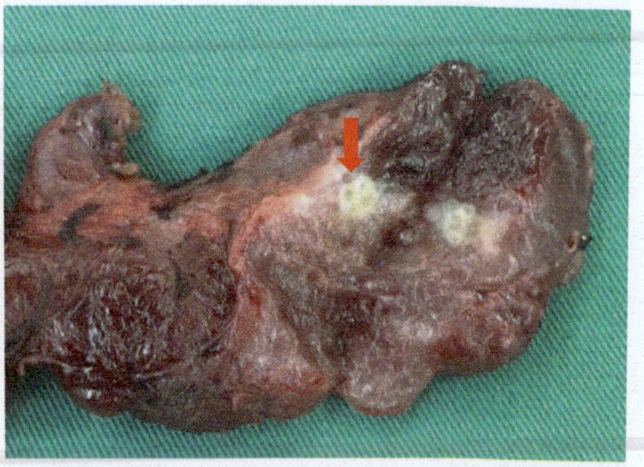

Fig. 7.22 Gross specimen of Case 32. A 0.7-cm gray and white nodule with ill-defined margin, the nodule is close to capsule

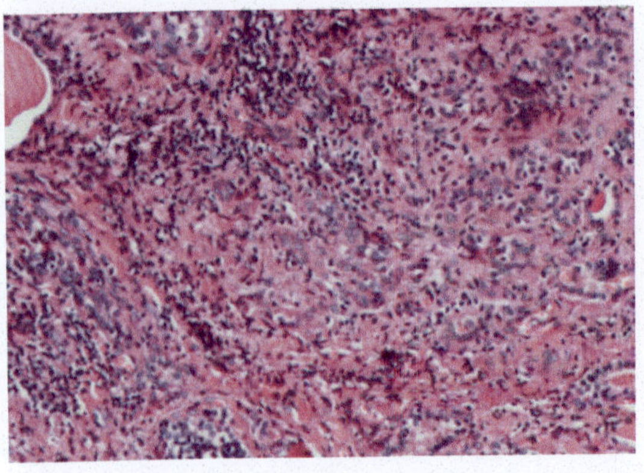

Fig. 7.20 Pathological diagnosis of Case 32: (right) Papillary thyroid microcarcinoma (0.5 cm)

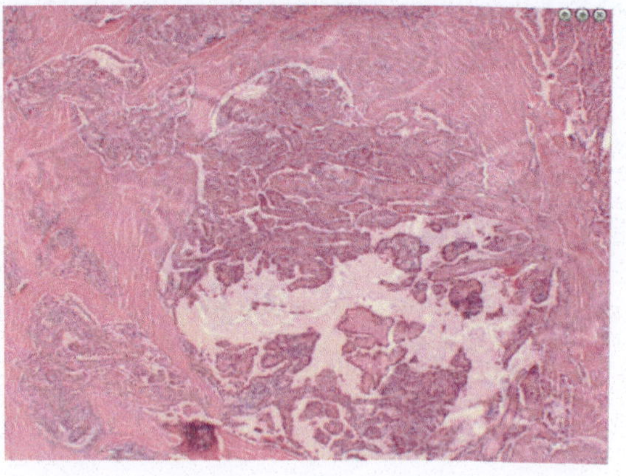

Fig. 7.23 Pathological diagnosis of Case 32: Papillary thyroid microcarcinoma

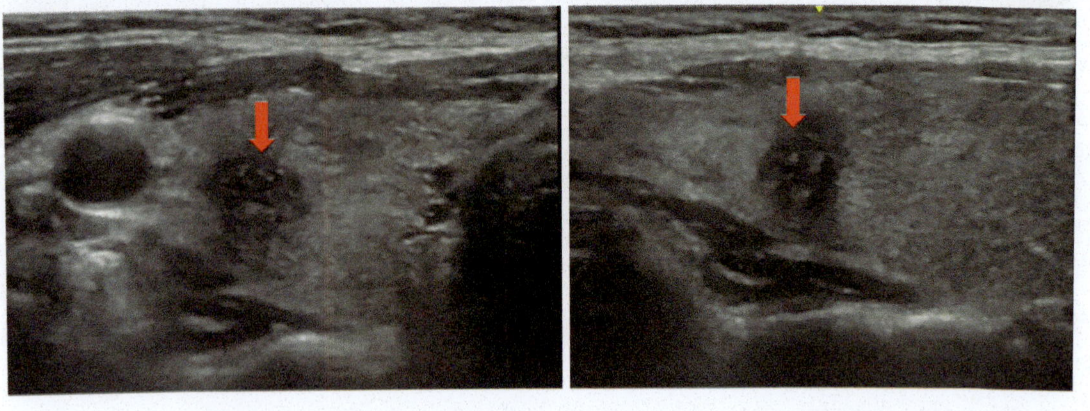

Fig. 7.21 Preoperative ultrasonic reevaluation of Case 32. A taller than wide hypoechoic nodule in the right lobe

Preoperative ultrasound evaluation: Fig. 7.24

Gross specimen and pathological diagnosis: Figs. 7.25 and 7.26

Case 35: Calcification

Clinical information: A 35-year-old male patient was detected with thyroid nodule for three years. Specialized physical examination: A tough nodule about 1.0 cm in the left thyroid lobe could be palpated, which moves up and down along with swallowing.

Preoperative ultrasound evaluation: Figs. 7.27 and 7.28

Gross specimen and pathological diagnosis: Figs. 7.28 and 7.29.

Case 36: Calcification

Clinical information: A 53-year-old male patient was detected with left thyroid nodule for 10 days. Specialized physical examination: A tough nodule about 1.0 cm in the left thyroid lobe could be palpated, which moves up and down along with swallowing.

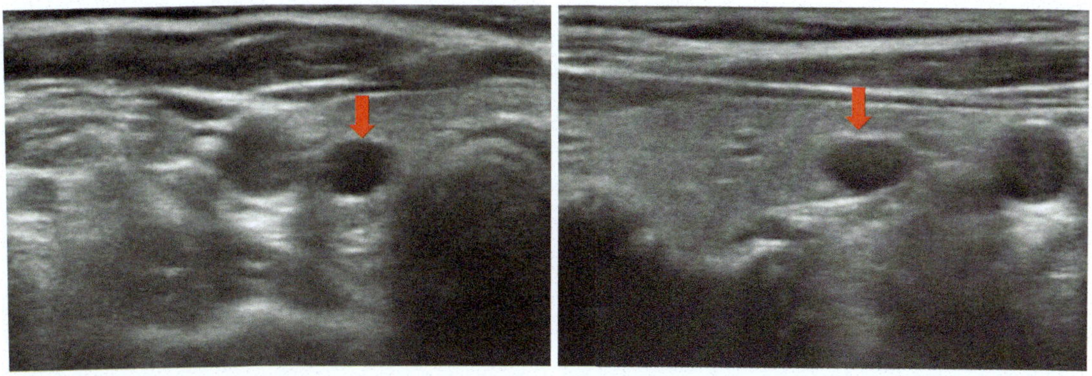

Fig. 7.24 Preoperative ultrasonic reevaluation of Case 34. A hypoechoic nodule in the right lobe with clear margin

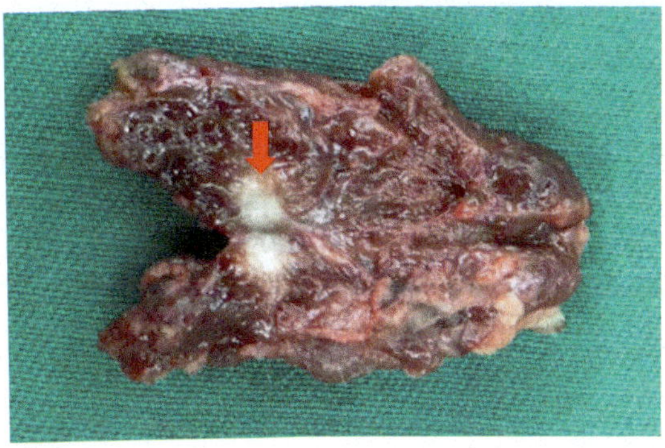

Fig. 7.25 Gross specimen of Case 34. A 0.4-cm gray and white nodule

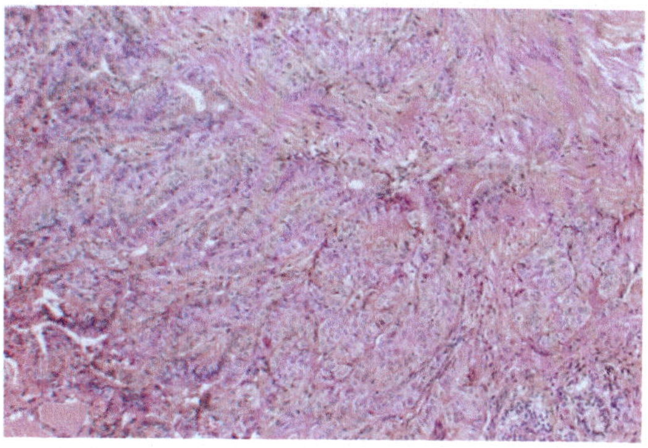

Fig. 7.26 Pathological diagnosis of Case 34 Papillary thyroid microcarcinoma

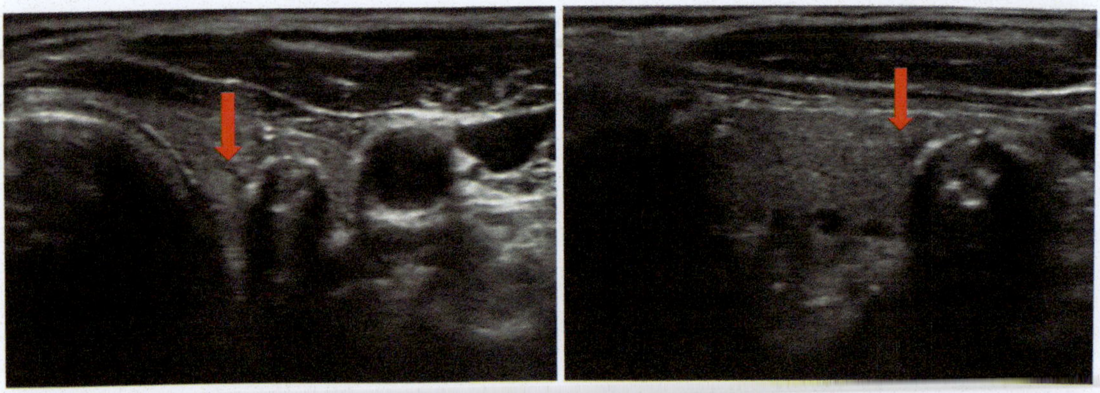

Fig. 7.27 Preoperative ultrasonic reevaluation of Case 34. A hypoechoic nodule in the right lobe with clear margin

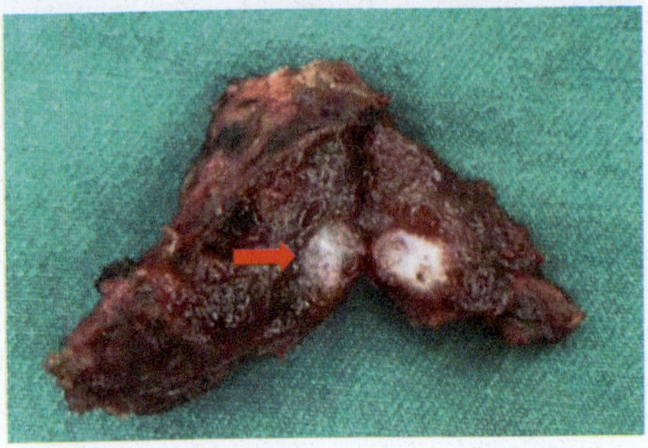

Fig. 7.28 Gross specimen of Case 35. A 0.7-cm gray and white nodule

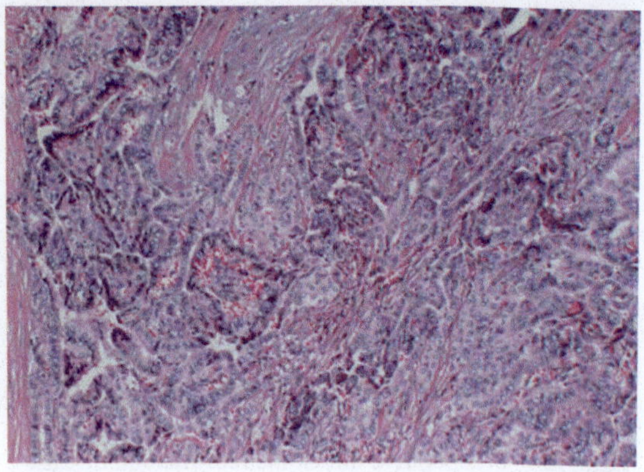

Fig. 7.29 Pathological diagnosis of Case 35 Papillary thyroid microcarcinoma

Ultrasonic information: Fig. 7.30

Preoperative ultrasound evaluation: Fig. 7.31

Gross specimen and pathological diagnosis: Figs. 7.22, 7.23, 7.32, and 7.33.

Case 37: Calcification

Clinical information: A 49-year-old male patient was detected with bilateral thyroid nodules for one week. T3, T4, and TSH levels were normal.

Ultrasonic information: Fig. 7.34

Preoperative ultrasound evaluation: Fig. 7.35

Gross specimen and pathological diagnosis: Figs. 7.36 and 7.37

Case 38: Calcification, Taller than Wide

Clinical information: A 50-year-old male patient was detected with thyroid nodules for 2 days. T3, T4, and TSH levels were normal.

Ultrasonic information: Fig. 7.38

Preoperative ultrasound evaluation: Fig. 7.39

Gross specimen and pathological diagnosis: Figs. 7.40 and 7.41.

Case 39: Calcification, Taller than Wide

Clinical information: A 56-year-old male patient was detected with bilateral thyroid nodule for two

Sonographic findings:

Size and shape were normal on thyroid transverse view. A taller than wide 1.01 cm × 0.66 cm hypoechoic foci with clear margin and irregular shape was observed in the of right lobe. The nodule contained uneven echogenicity and punctate hyperechogenicity inside, one of which was 0.15 cm in size. Several echofree spaces in the parenchyma of left lobe with regular shape and clear margin, one of which was 0.35 cm × 0.28 cm in size. Hypoechoic foci around the echofree space could be detected with acoustic shadowing behind.

CDFI: Patchy blood flow signals were observed in the hypoechoic nodule.

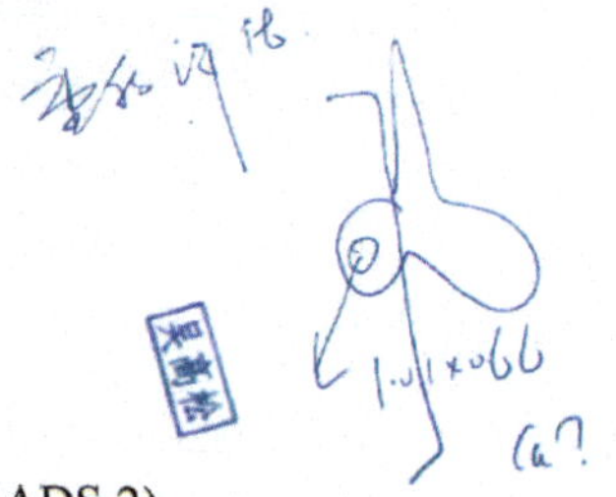

Sonographic indicates:

Solid nodule in the right lobe with calcification (TI-RADS 4b)

Cystic nodules in the left lobe (Concentrated colloid cysts) (TI-RADS 2)

Fig. 7.30 Sonographic report of Case 36

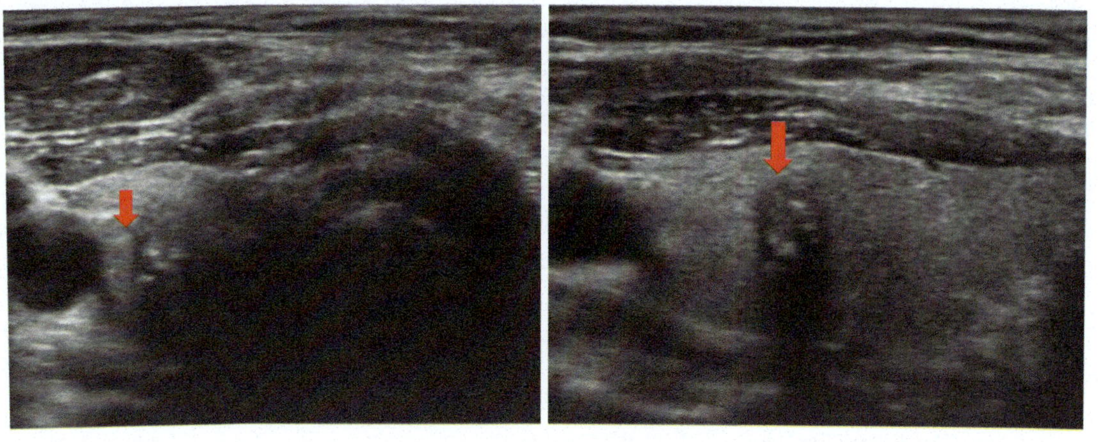

Fig. 7.31 Preoperative ultrasonic reevaluation of Case 36. A hypoechoic nodule with punctate hyperechoic foci inside

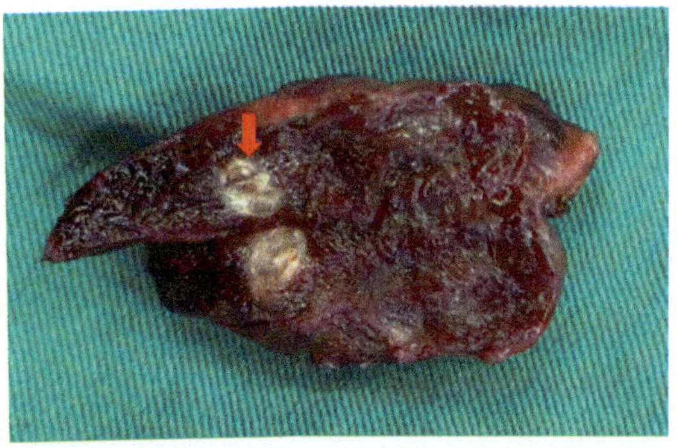

Fig. 7.32 Gross specimen of Case 36. A 0.7-cm gray and white nodule with clear margin

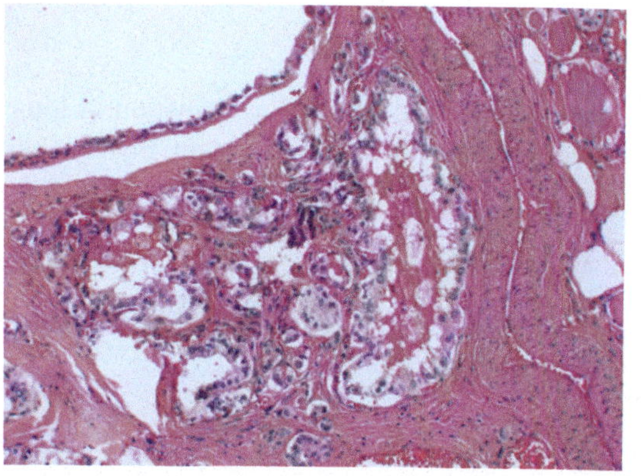

Fig. 7.33 Pathological diagnosis of Case 36 Papillary thyroid microcarcinoma

Ultrasonic images:

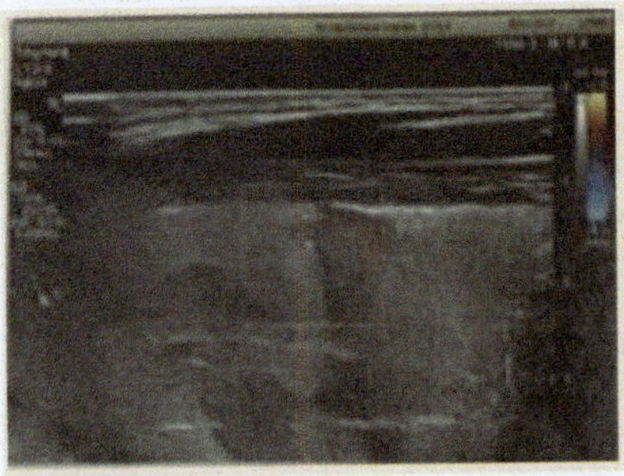

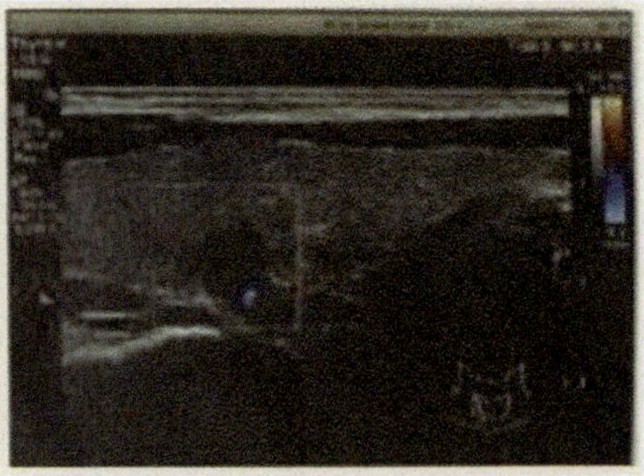

Sonographic findings:

Size and shape were normal on thyroid transverse view. A 0.5 cm × 0.5 cm hypoechoic solid nodule with clear margin and uneven echogenicity inside in the middle upper of left lobe. This nodule was in horizontal and contained hyperechoic foci inside. A 0.5 cm × 0.5 cm hypoechoic solid nodule with clear margin and uneven echogenicity inside in the middle of right lobes.

No abnormal echogenicity was detected in the bilateral parathyroid gland area.

CDFI: Patchy blood flow signals were observed in the hypoechoic nodule.

Several hypoechoic solid nodules with clear margin were detected in the level II, III, IV, VI, one of which was 1.5 cm × 0. 4cm in the left, 1.9 cm × 0.6 cm in the right.

CDFI: Blood flow signals were observed in the aforementioned nodules.

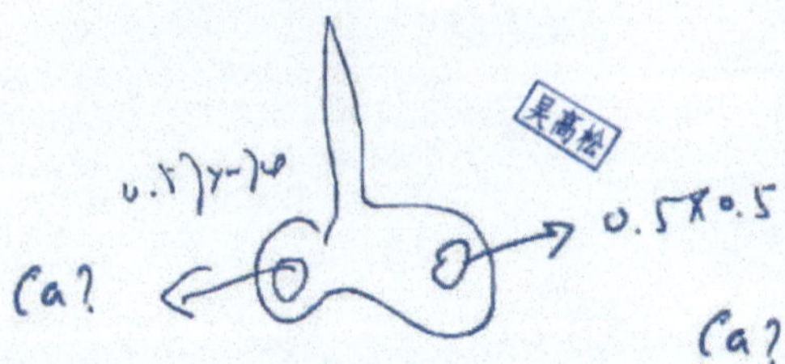

Sonographic indicates

Solid nodule in the left lobe with coarse calcification (ACR TI-RADS 4b)

Solid nodule in the right lobe (ACR TI-RADS 4b)

Fig. 7.34 Sonographic report of Case 37

years. Specialized physical examination: A tough nodule about 2.0 cm in the right thyroid lobe could be palpated, which moves up and down along with swallowing. FT3: 5.02 pmol/L (3.21–6.5 pmol/L), FT4: 16.47pmol/L (10.22–21.88 pmol/L), TSH: 2.25 μU/mL (0.3–4.6 μU/mL), Anti-Tg: 34 U/mL (0–72 U/mL), A-TPO 489 U/mL ↑ (0–16 U/mL).

Ultrasonic information: Fig. 7.42

Preoperative ultrasound evaluation: Fig. 7.43

Gross specimen and pathological diagnosis: Figs. 7.44 and 7.45

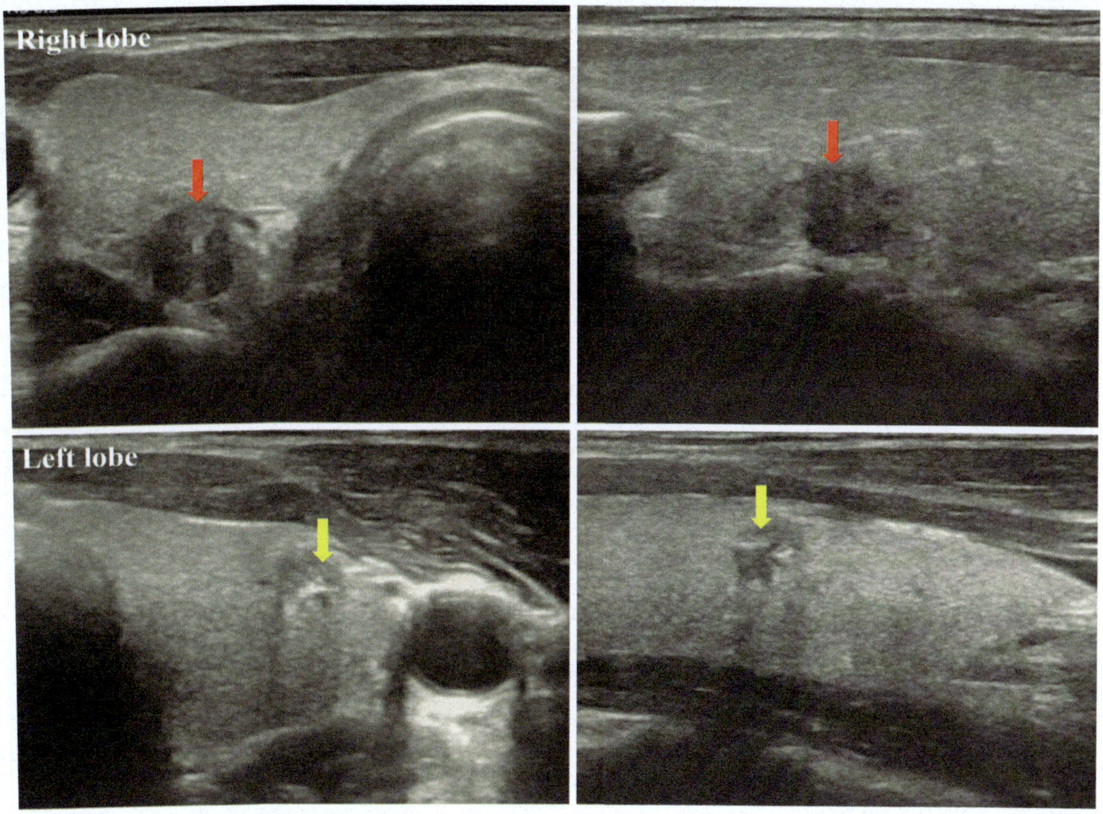

Fig. 7.35 Preoperative ultrasonic reevaluation of Case 37. Shape of the right hyperechoic nodule tend to be spherical, hyperechogenic foci was observed in the left nodule

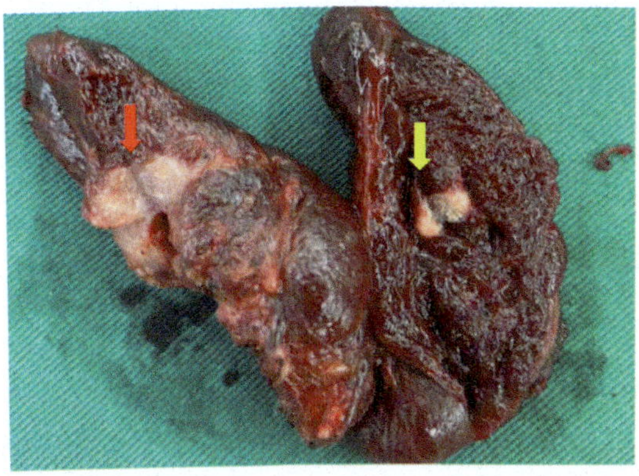

Fig. 7.36 Gross specimen of Case 37. White nodules in the bilateral thyroid lobes

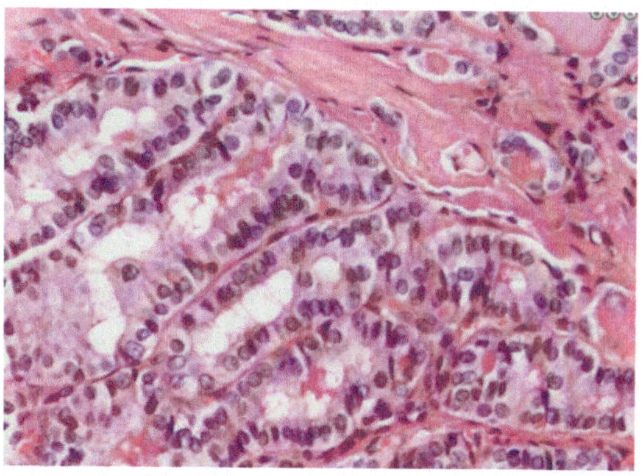

Fig. 7.37 Pathological diagnosis of Case 37 Papillary thyroid microcarcinoma

Ultrasonic images:

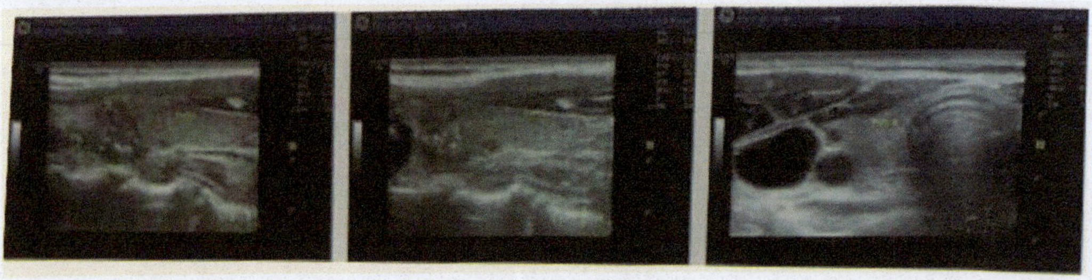

Sonographic findings:

Thyroid scan

Size and shape were normal on thyroid transverse view. The echogenicity of parenchyma was uneven.

Left lobe:

A taller than wide hypoechoic 1.1 cm × 1.4 cm nodule in the superior pole with ill-defined margin, irregular shape and uneven echogenicity inside (no blood flow).

Several sightly low hypoechoic masses with ill-defined margin and uneven echogenicity inside were detected in the middle of the left lobe one of which was 0.4 cm × 0.4 cm in size.

Right lobe:

Several anechoic masses with clear margin and increased echogenicity behind, one of which was 0.3 cm × 0.2 cm in size.

Sonographic indicates:

Hypoechoic nodule in the left lobe with calcification (TI-RADS 5)

Sightly low hypoechoic nodule in the left lobe with calcification (TI-RADS 3)

Anechoic mass in the right lobe (colloid cyst? TI-RADS 2)

Fig. 7.38 Sonographic report of Case 38

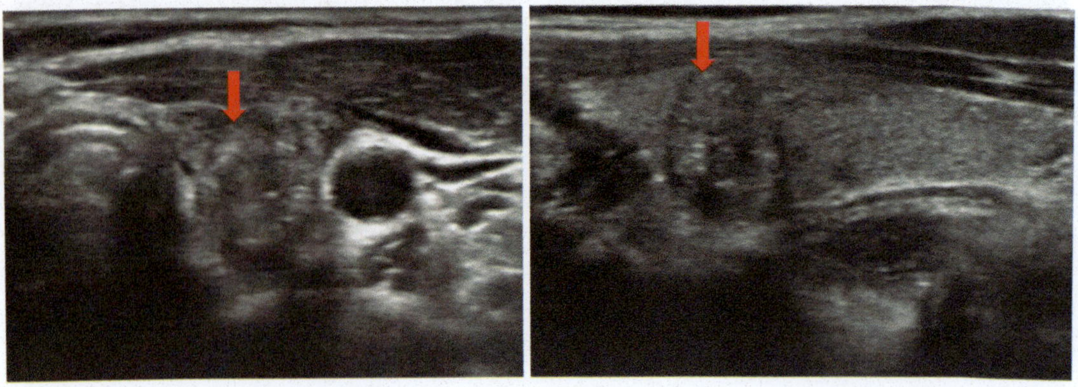

Fig. 7.39 Preoperative ultrasonic reevaluation of Case 38. Calcification, taller than wide, punctate echogenic foci inside

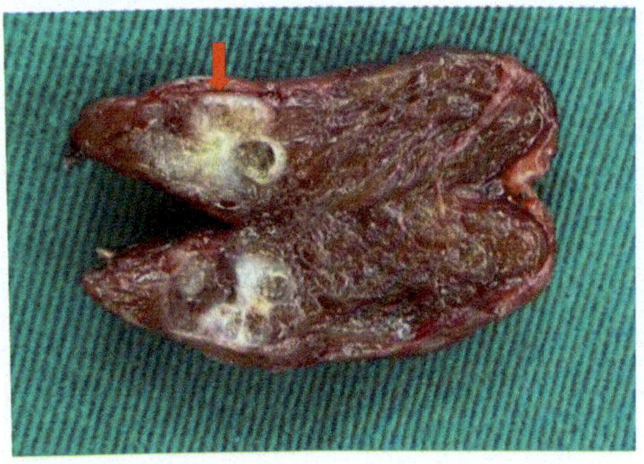

Fig. 7.40 Gross specimen of Case 37. A 1.0-cm gray-white-gray-yellow nodule

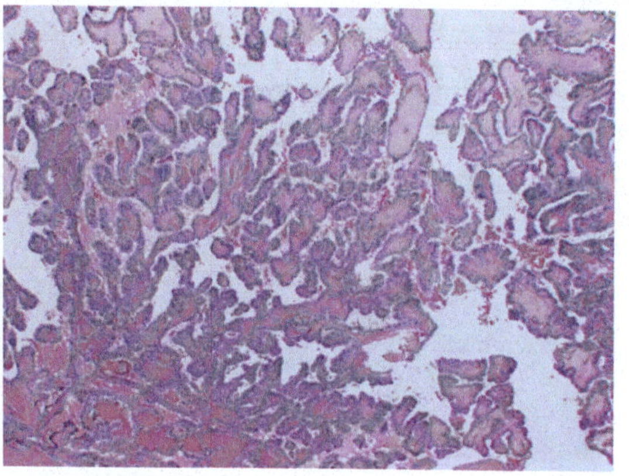

Fig. 7.41 Pathological diagnosis of Case 38 Papillary thyroid carcinoma

Ultrasonic images:

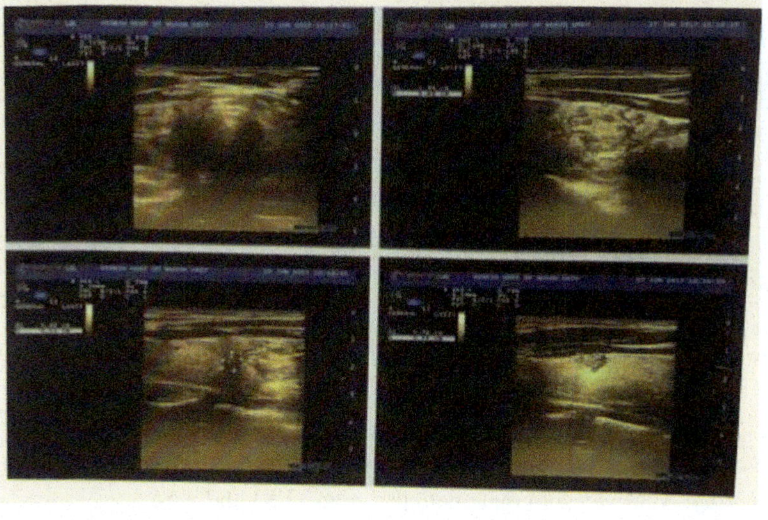

Sonographic findings:

Size and shape were normal on thyroid transverse view with integrity capsule. The echogenicity of parenchyma was uniform. Several hypoechoic masses with clear margin and uneven echogenicity inside were detected in the right lobe, one of which was 2.0 cm × 1.7 cm in size. A taller than wide 0.7 cm × 0.5 cm very low hypoechoic nodule with ill-defined margin was detected in the right lobe. A taller than wide 0.8 cm × 0.5 cm mixed echogenicity nodule with clear margin was detected in the left lobe.

CDFI: No blood flow signals were observed in thyroid gland and few blood flow signals were observed in the hypoechoic foci.

Sonographic indicates:

Very low hypoechoic nodule in the right lobe (TI-RADS 4c)

Hypoechoic nodule in the right lobe (TI-RADS 3)

Mixed echogenicity nodule in the left lobe (TI-RADS 3)

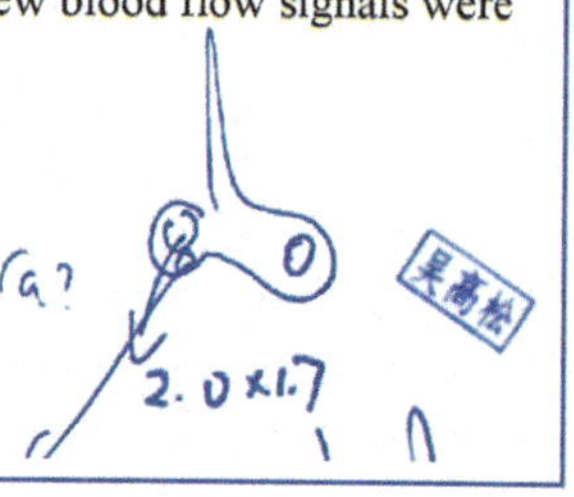

Fig. 7.42 Sonographic report of Case 39

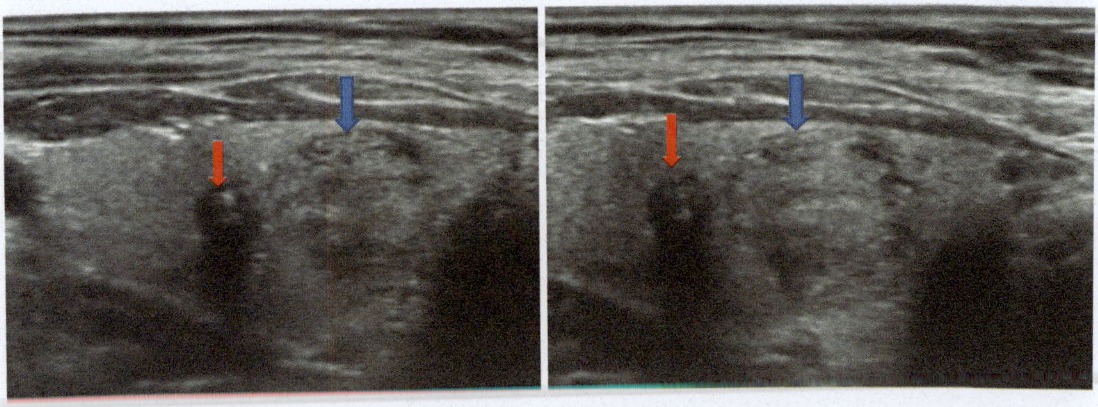

Fig. 7.43 Preoperative ultrasonic reevaluation of Case 39. A taller than wide 0.7 cm hypoechoic nodule with punctate hyperechogenicity inside, and an anechoic nodule was alongside

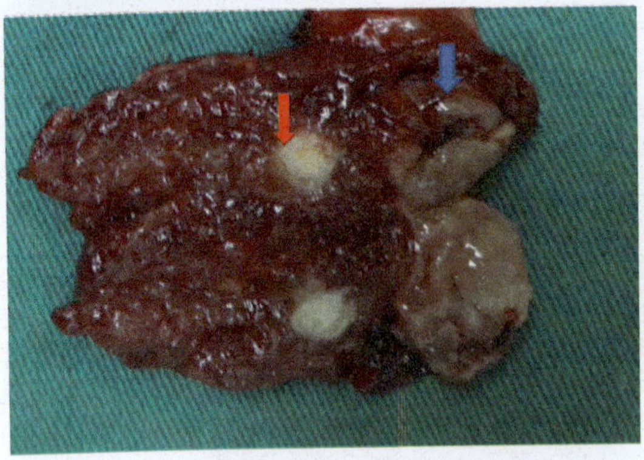

Fig. 7.44 Gross specimen of Case 39. A 0.7-cm gray-white-gray-yellow nodule and a Gray-white translucent nodule

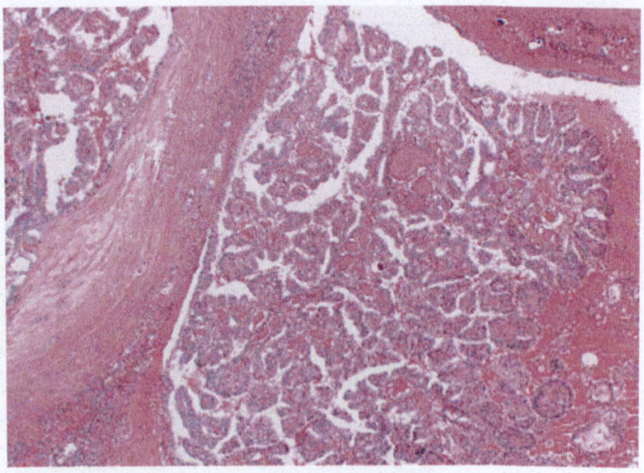

Fig. 7.45 Pathological diagnosis of Case 39 Papillary thyroid microcarcinoma

Case 40

Clinical information: A 30-year-old male patient was detected with thyroid nodules for one week. T3, T4, and TSH levels were normal.

Ultrasonic information: Fig. 7.46

Preoperative ultrasound evaluation: Fig. 7.47

Gross specimen and pathological diagnosis: Figs. 7.48 and 7.49.

Case 41

Clinical information: A 43-year-old male patient was detected with thyroid nodules for one week. T3, T4, and TSH levels were normal.

Ultrasonic information: Figs. 7.50 and 7.51.

Preoperative ultrasound evaluation: Fig. 7.52

Gross specimen and pathological diagnosis: Figs. 7.53 and 7.54.

Case 42

Clinical information: A 51-year-old female patient was detected with thyroid nodules for one week. T3, T4, and TSH levels were normal.

Ultrasonic information: Fig. 7.55

Preoperative ultrasound evaluation: Fig. 7.56

Gross specimen and pathological diagnosis: Figs. 7.50, 7.51, and 7.57.

Case 43

Clinical information: A 37-year-old female patient was detected with left thyroid nodule for

Ultrasonic images:

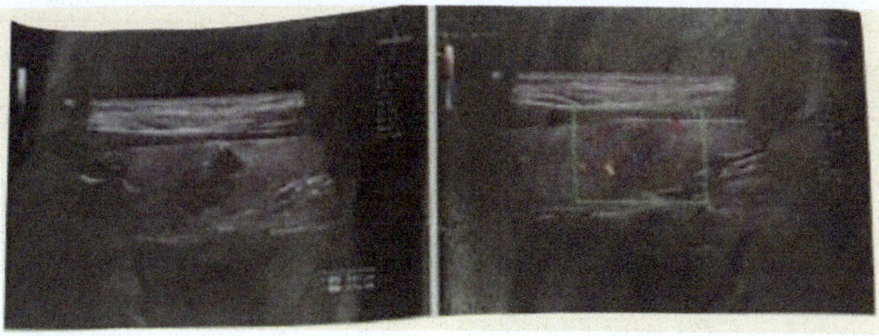

Sonographic findings:

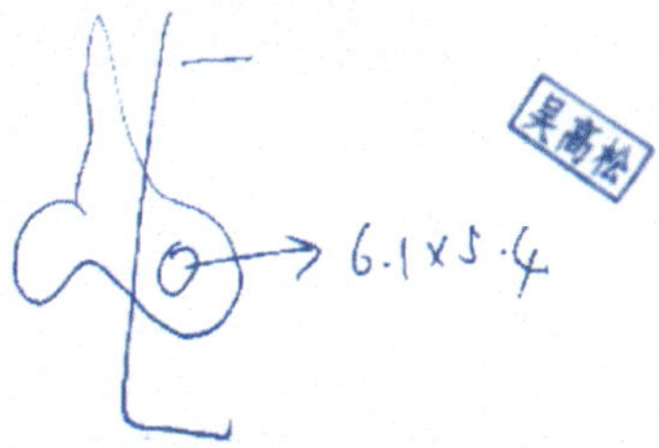

Thyroid scan

Left lobe: 48 mm × 18 mm × 15 mm.

Right lobe: 46 mm × 17 mm × 15 mm.

Isthmus: anteroposterior diameter is 0.2 cm.

A 6.1 mm × 5.4 mm hypoechoic nodule with clear margin and irregular shape was detected in the middle of left lobe.

CDFI: Irregular course blood flow signals were observed in the hypoechoic nodule.

Sonographic indicates:

Solid nodule in the left lobe with calcification

Fig. 7.46 Sonographic report of Case 40

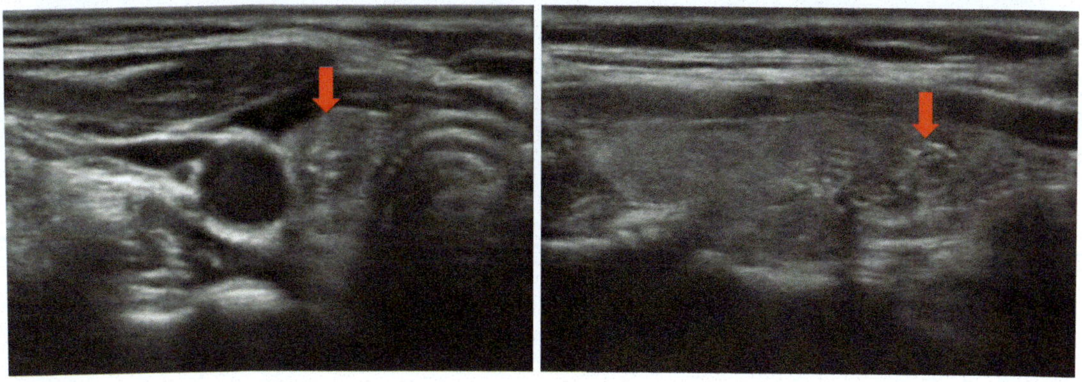

Fig. 7.47 Preoperative ultrasonic reevaluation of Case 40. Obvious punctate hyperechogenicity were observed in the nodule

two months. Specialized physical examination: A tough nodule about 3.0 cm in the right thyroid lobe could be palpated, which moves up and down along with swallowing.

Ultrasonic information: Fig. 7.58.

Preoperative ultrasound evaluation: Fig. 7.59.

Gross specimen and pathological diagnosis: Figs. 7.60 and 7.61.

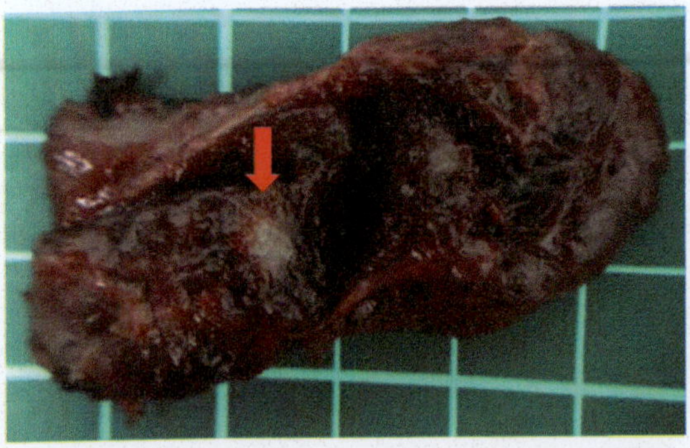

Fig. 7.48 Gross specimen of Case 39. A 0.3 cm × 0.2 cm gray-white hard nodule

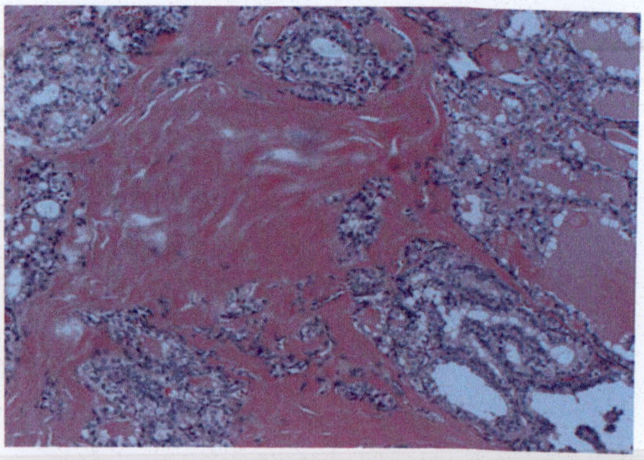

Fig. 7.49 Pathological diagnosis of Case 39 Papillary thyroid microcarcinoma

Ultrasonic images:

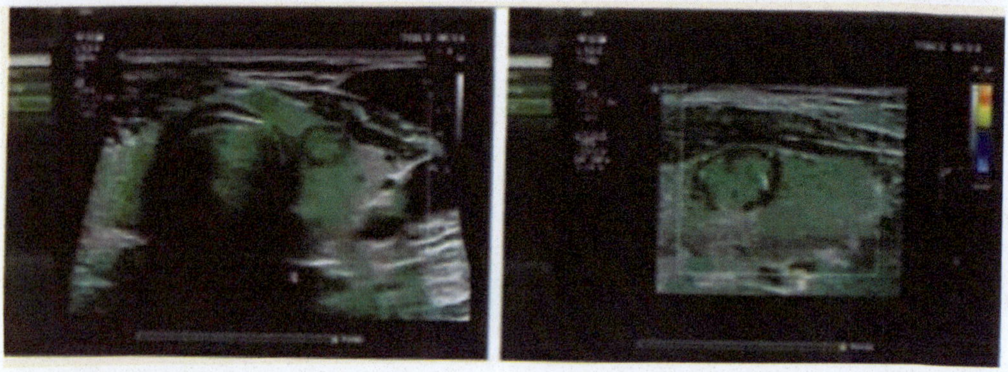

Sonographic findings:

Thyroid scan

Left lobe: 4.3 cm × 1.5 cm × 1.8 cm.

Right lobe: 4.4 cm × 1.4 cm × 1.6 cm.

Isthmus: anteroposterior diameter is 0.28 cm. Size and shape were abnormal on right thyroid lobe. The echogenicity of parenchyma is uniform. No nodules were detected in the right lobe.

A 1.0 cm × 0.7 cm hypoechoic nodule with clear margin, regular shape and coarse calcification inside was detected in the left lobe.

CDFI: Blood flow signals were observed in the left nodule.

Sonographic indicates:

Hypoechoic nodule in the left lobe with calcification (TI-RADS 4a)

Fig. 7.50 Sonographic report of Case 41 (1)

Ultrasonic images:

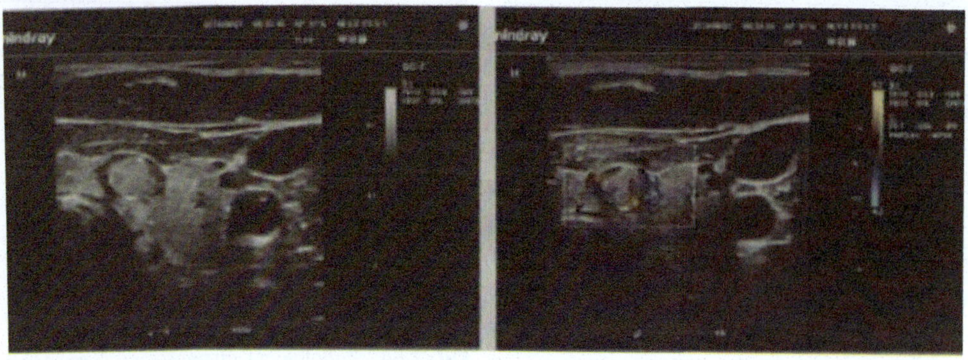

Sonographic findings:

Thyroid scan

The shape of the lobe was plump, with uneven echogenicity in the parenchyma.

Left lobe:

An isoechoic 0.94 cm × 0.64 cm nodule with ill-defined margin and irregular shape was detected in the middle superior of left lobe close to isthmus. The nodule contained uneven echogenicity and scattered punctate hyperechogenicity inside.

Right lobe:

No obvious echogenicity was detected.

Bilateral neck scan:

There is no echogenicity of enlarged lymph node close to the large blood vessels in both sides of the neck.

Sonographic indicates:

Isoechoic nodule in the left lobe with microcalcification (TI-RADS 4b)

Fig. 7.51 Sonographic report of Case 41 (2)

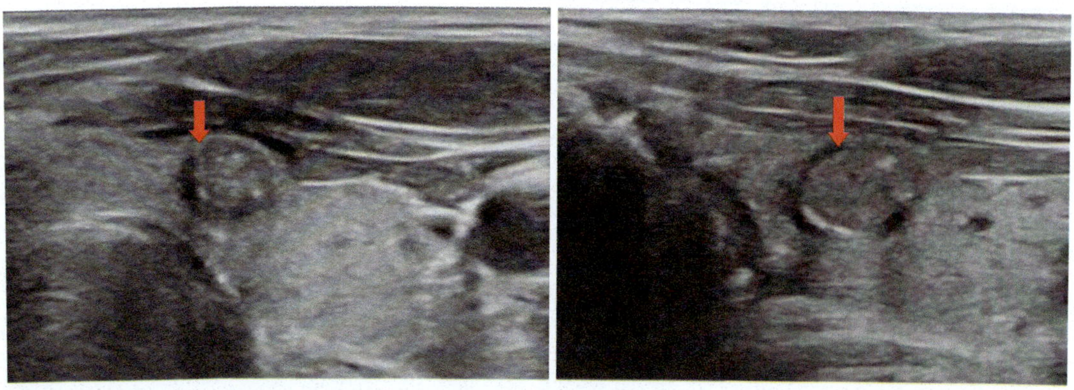

Fig. 7.52 Preoperative ultrasonic reevaluation of Case 41. Punctate hyperechogenicity in the nodule

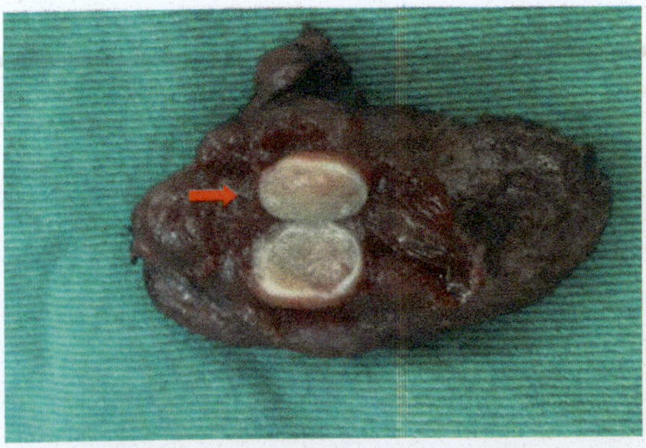

Fig. 7.53 Gross specimen of Case 41. A gray-white nodule

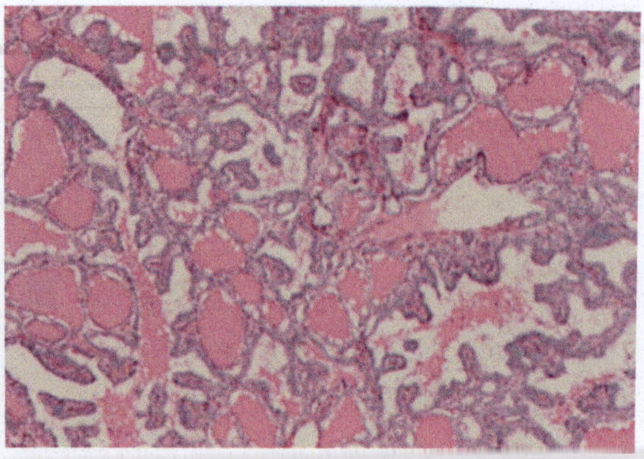

Fig. 7.54 Pathological diagnosis of Case 41 Papillary thyroid carcinoma

Sonographic findings:

Thyroid scan

Left lobe: 4.1 cm × 0.8 cm × 1.3 cm.

Right lobe: 3.8 cm × 0.9 cm × 1.2 cm.

Isthmus: anteroposterior diameter is 0.24 cm.

Size and shape were normal on thyroid transverse view. The echogenicity of parenchyma was uneven. A 0.3 cm × 0.1 cm anechoic nodule with clear margin and increased echogenicity behind was detected in the left lobe. A 1.8 cm × 1.1 cm hypoechoic nodule with ill-defined margin and uneven echogenicity inside was detected in the right lobe. A 0.3 cm × 0.4 cm hypoechoic nodule with ill-defined margin and uneven echogenicity inside was detected in right lobe, hyperechoic foci were observed in the nodule.

CDFI: No blood flow signals were observed in the above nodules.

Sonographic indicates:

Hypoechoic nodule in the right lobe (TI-RADS 4b)

Anechoic nodule in the left lobe (TI-RADS 2)

Fig. 7.55 Sonographic report of Case 42

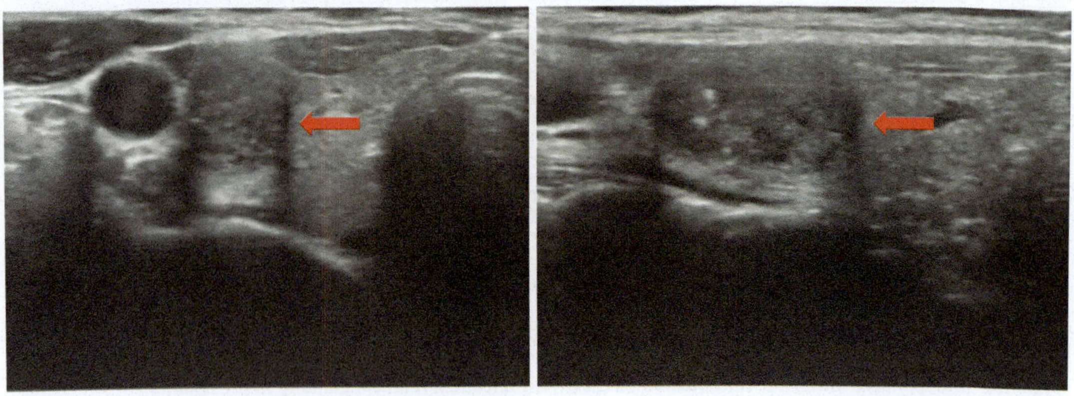

Fig. 7.56 Preoperative ultrasonic reevaluation of Case 42. Punctate hyperechogenicity in the irregular nodule

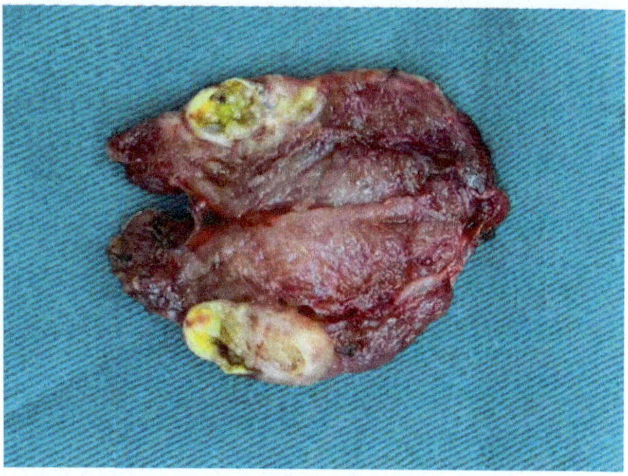

Fig. 7.57 Gross specimen of Case 42. A gray-white nodule was observed, pathological diagnosis was papillary thyroid carcinoma

Ultrasonic images:

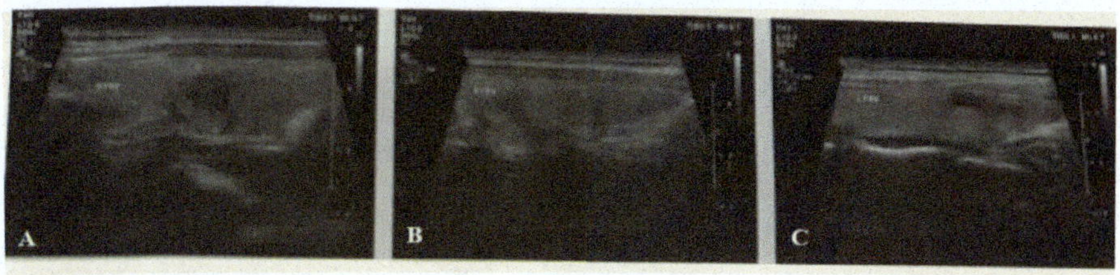

Sonographic findings:

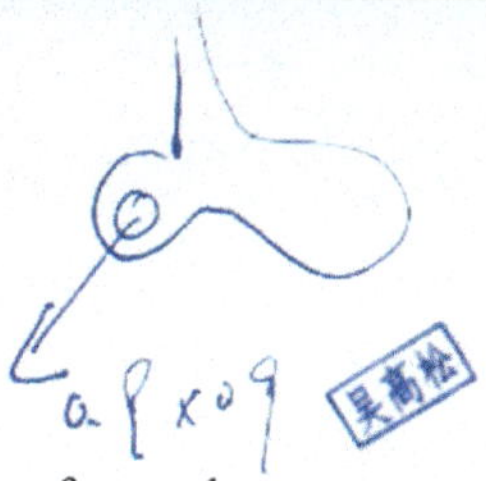

Thyroid scan

Left lobe: 4.6 cm × 1.5 cm × 1.2 cm.

Right lobe: 5.0 cm × 1.5 cm × 1.1 cm.

Isthmus: anteroposterior diameter is 0.24 cm.

Size and shape of the thyroid gland were normal. The echogenicity of parenchyma was uneven. A 0.9 cm × 0.9 cm sightly low hypoechoic nodule with clear margin, regular shape, and uneven echogenicity inside was detected in the middle dorsal of right lobe. This nodule contained scattered punctate hyperechogenicity, comet-tail sign behind and hypoechoic acoustic halo surroundingly, no colored flow signals were observed (A).

A 0.7 cm × 0.7 cm sightly low hypoechoic nodule with ill-defined margin, regular shape, and uneven echogenicity inside was detected in the middle inferior of right lobe (B) Colored flow signals were observed.

A 0.5 cm × 0.3 cm mixed echoic nodule with clear margin and uneven echogenicity inside was detected in inferior of left lobe, no colored flow signals were observed (C). Several anechoic areas with clear margin and increased echogenicity behind were observed in the left lobe, no colored flow signals were observed, one of which was 0.6cm× 0.3cm in size.

Sonographic indicates:

Sightly low hypoechoic nodule in the middle dorsal of right lobe (TI-RADS 4a)

Sightly low hypoechoic nodule in the middle inferior of right lobe (TI-RADS 3)

Cyst-solid mixed nodule echoic in inferior of left lobe (TI-RADS 3).

Cystic nodule in the left lobe (TI-RADS 2).

Fig. 7.58 Sonographic report of Case 43

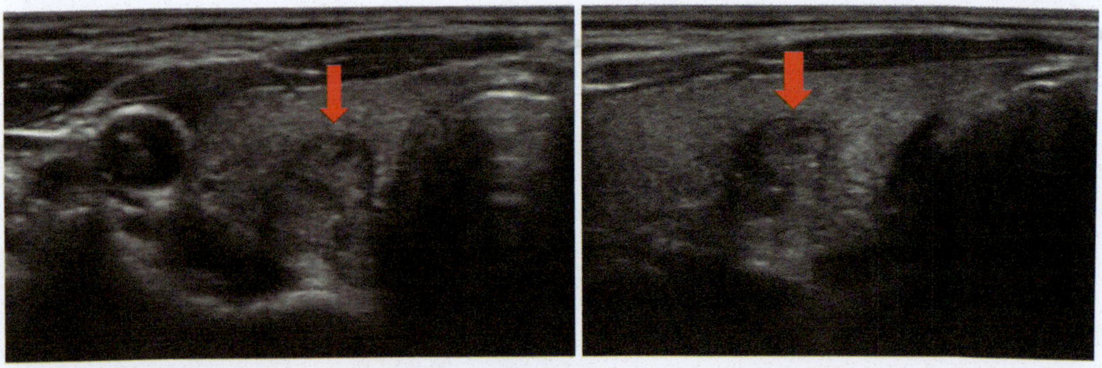

Fig. 7.59 Preoperative ultrasonic reevaluation of Case 42. A 0.9 cm × 0.9 cm hypoechoic nodule with an irregular shape and punctate hyperechogenicity surrounded by hypoechoic foci

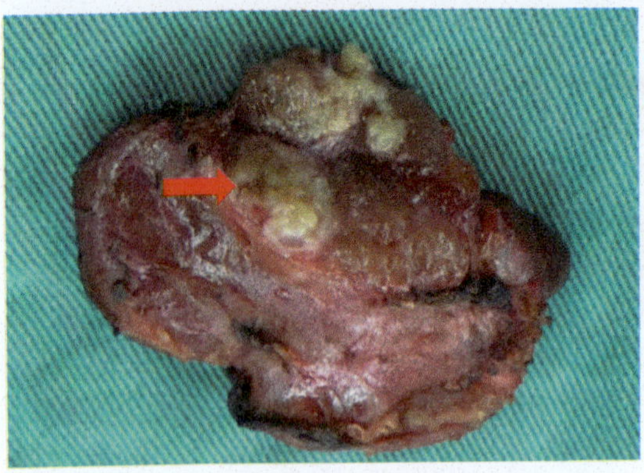

Fig. 7.60 Gross specimen of Case 43. A 0.7 cm gray-yellow nodule

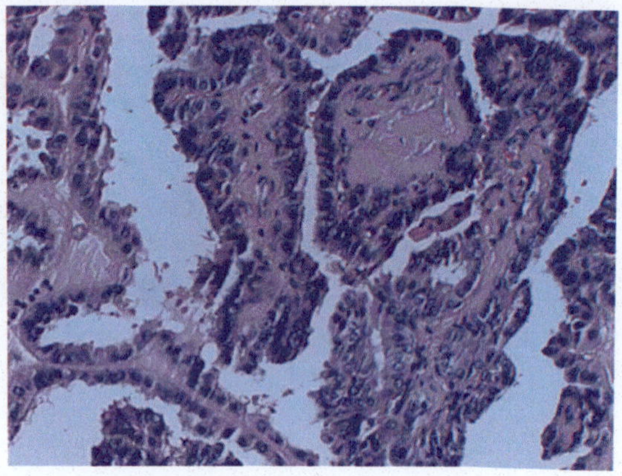

Fig. 7.61 Pathological diagnosis of Case 43 Papillary thyroid microcarcinoma

7.2 Category 2 TI-RADS 4a or 3 Thyroid Nodules Need to Be Evaluated Carefully

Case 44

Clinical information: A 57-year-old female patient was detected with thyroid nodules for one month. T3, T4, and TSH levels were normal.

Ultrasonic information: Figs. 7.62 and 7.63.

Preoperative ultrasound evaluation: Fig. 7.64

Gross specimen and pathological diagnosis: Figs. 7.65 and 7.66.

Case 45

Clinical information: A 63-year-old female patient was detected with thyroid nodule for one week. Specialized physical examination: A tough nodule about 1.0 cm in the right thyroid lobe could be palpated, which moves up and down along with swallowing.

Ultrasonic information: Fig. 7.67.

Preoperative ultrasound evaluation: Fig. 7.68.

Gross specimen and pathological diagnosis: Figs. 7.69 and 7.70.

Ultrasonic images:

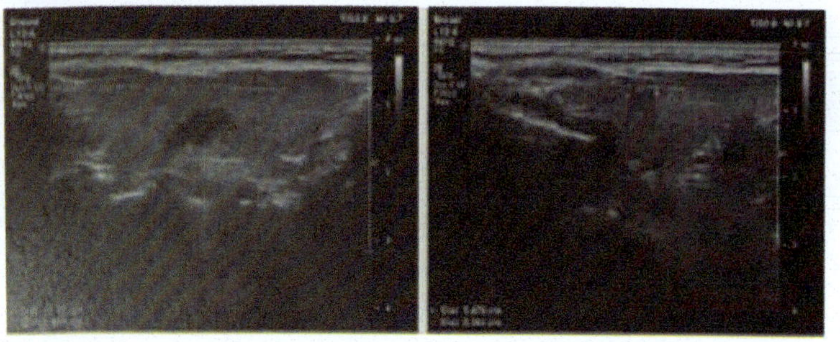

Sonographic findings:

Size and shape of the thyroid gland were normal. The echogenicity of parenchyma was uneven. Two mixed echoic areas (hypoechoic or anechoic) with clear margin and uneven echogenicity inside was detected in the right lobe, one of which was 1.4 cm × 0.8 cm in size. A 0.5 cm × 0.4 cm mixed echoic nodule (hypoechoic or anechoic) with clear margin and uneven echogenicity inside was detected in the left lobe. Two mixed echoic areas (hypoechoic or anechoic) with clear margin and uneven echogenicity inside was detected in left lobe, one of which was 0.3 cm × 0.2 cm in size.

No significantly enlarged lymph nodes were observed in the bilateral neck

CDFI: Blood flow signals were observed in the mixed echoic nodules.

Sonographic indicates:

Solid nodule in the right lobe (TI-RADS 4a)

Cyst-solid mixed nodule in the bilateral lobes (TI-RADS 3)

Solid nodule in the left lobe (TI-RADS 3)

Fig. 7.62 Sonographic report of Case 44 (1)

Case 46

Clinical information: A 48-year-old female patient was detected with thyroid nodules for one week without clinical symptoms. T3, T4, and TSH levels were normal.

Ultrasonic information: Fig. 7.71.

Preoperative ultrasound evaluation: Fig. 7.72.

Gross specimen and pathological diagnosis: Figs. 7.73, 7.74, and 7.75.

Case 47

Clinical information: A 48-year-old female patient was detected with thyroid nodules for one week without clinical symptoms. T3, T4, and TSH levels were normal.

Ultrasonic information: Figs. 7.76 and 7.77.

Preoperative ultrasound evaluation: Fig. 7.78

Gross specimen and pathological diagnosis: Figs. 7.79 and 7.80.

Ultrasonic images:

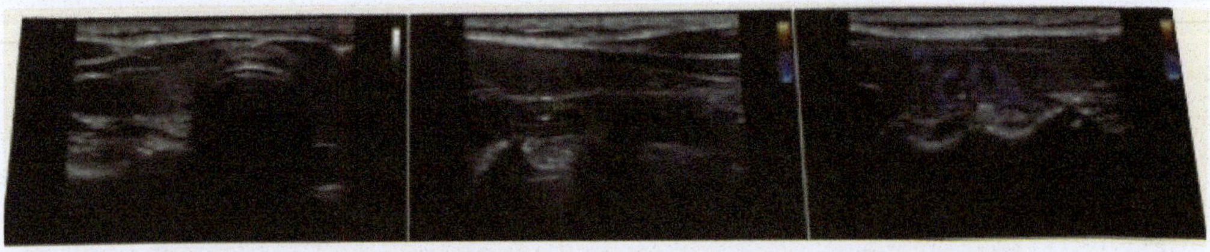

Sonographic findings:

Thyroid scan

Left lobe: 3.8cm× 0.9cm× 0.7cm.

Right lobe: 4.5cm× 1.1cm× 1.1cm.

Isthmus: anteroposterior diameter is 0.16 cm.

Size and shape of the thyroid gland were normal. The echogenicity of parenchyma was uneven. A 0.5 cm × 0.2 cm hypoechoic nodule with ill-defined margin and uneven echogenicity inside was detected in the left lobe.

A 1.2 cm × 0.6 cm × 0.6 cm hypoechoic nodule with ill-defined margin and uneven echogenicity inside was detected in the right lobe. Punctate hyperechogenicity and comet-tail sign were observed.

A 0.3 cm × 0.3 cm hypoechoic nodule with clear margin and uneven echogenicity inside was detected in the isthmus of thyroid.

CDFI: Colored blood flow signals were observed in the hypoechoelocyle of the right lobe, arterial spectrum was detected, RI: 0.61.

Sonographic indicates:

Hypoechoic nodule with calcification in the right lobe (TI-RADS 4a)

Hypoechoic nodule in the left lobe and the isthmus of thyroid (TI-RADS 3)

Fig. 7.63 Sonographic report of Case 44 (2)

Case 48

Clinical information: A 39-year-old female patient was detected with thyroid nodules for three years without clinical symptoms. T3, T4, and TSH levels were normal.

Ultrasonic information: Fig. 7.81.

Preoperative ultrasound evaluation: Nodule 1 was a cyst-solid mixed nodule, mainly in cyst with punctate hyperechogenicity inside. Most partially cystic thyroid nodules(PCTN) result from degenerative changes in benign nodules. The malignant signs of PCTN often include eccentric and acute angle between the nodular sac wall and the solid part of the free edge, microcalcification in solid nodules, lobulated or irregular margin of solid nodules. The nodules are indistinct and infiltrated peripherally. There were abundant blood flows in the nodular attachments or solid parts, and abnormal lymph nodes are observed. Benign signs include concentric or

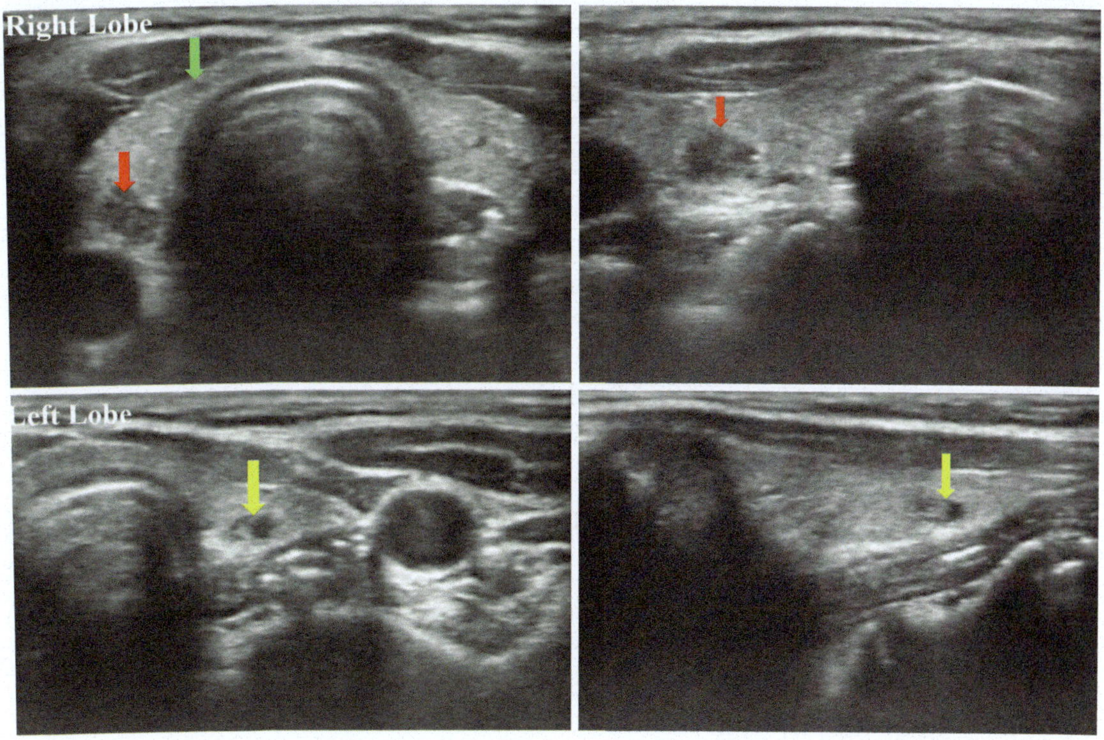

Fig. 7.64 Preoperative ultrasonic reevaluation of Case 44. Hypoechoic nodules with irregular shape and punctate hyperechogenicity in the right lobe (red arrow). Hypoechoic nodule in the right lobe (green arrow). Cyst-solid mixed nodules in the left lobe (yellow arrow)

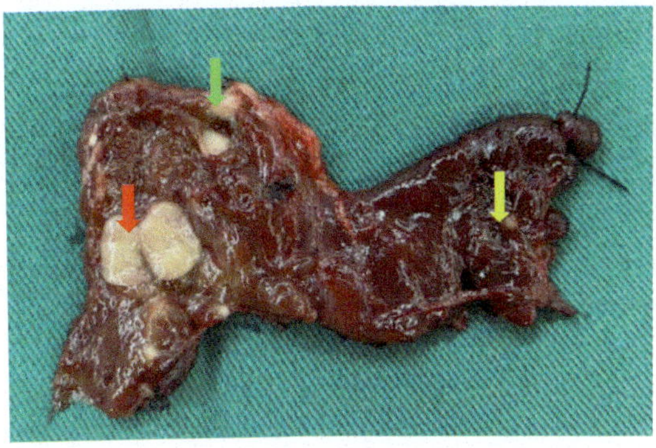

Fig. 7.65 Gross specimen of Case 44. Gray-white nodules 1.5 cm and 0.2 cm in size, were seen in the right lobe, 0.2 cm gray-white nodule in the left nodule

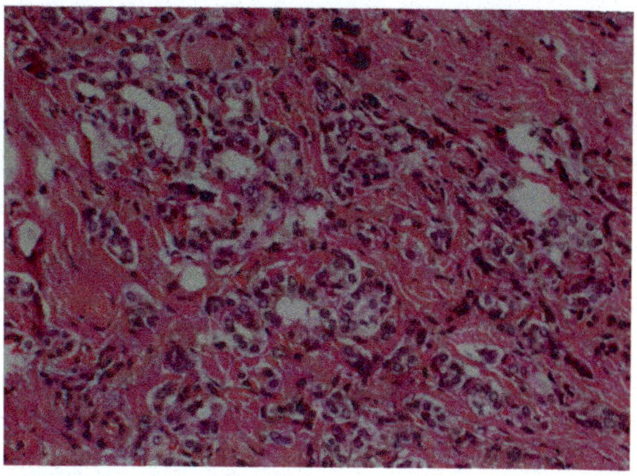

Fig. 7.66 Pathological diagnosis of Case 44 Bilateral papillary thyroid microcarcinoma

Sonographic findings:

Thyroid scan

Left lobe: 4.3 cm × 1.2 cm × 1.0 cm.

Right lobe: 5.2 cm × 1.8 cm × 1.5 cm.

Isthmus: anteroposterior diameter is 0.29 cm.

Size and shape of the thyroid gland were normal. The echogenicity of parenchyma was uneven. A 1.8 cm × 1.1 cm mixed echoic nodule with clear margin was detected in the right lobe. This nodule was mainly in hypoechogenicity with anechogenicity and punctate hyperechogenicity inside, and blood flow sign was observed.

Several hypoechoic nodules with ill-defined margin and blood flow sign inside was detected in the left lobe, one of which was 0.5 cm × 0.3 cm in size with acoustic shadowing behind.

Sonographic indicates:

Mixed echoic nodule in the right lobe (TI-RADS 4a)

Hypoechoic nodule in the left lobe (TI-RADS 3)

Calcification foci in the left lobe

Diffuse lesions of the thyroid gland

Fig. 7.67 Sonographic report of Case 45

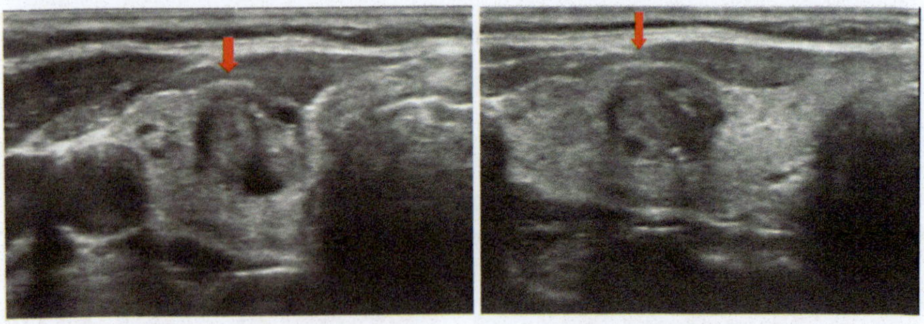

Fig. 7.68 Preoperative ultrasonic reevaluation of Case 45. Cyst-solid mixed nodule in the right lobe, mainly in solid, with punctate hyperechogenicity

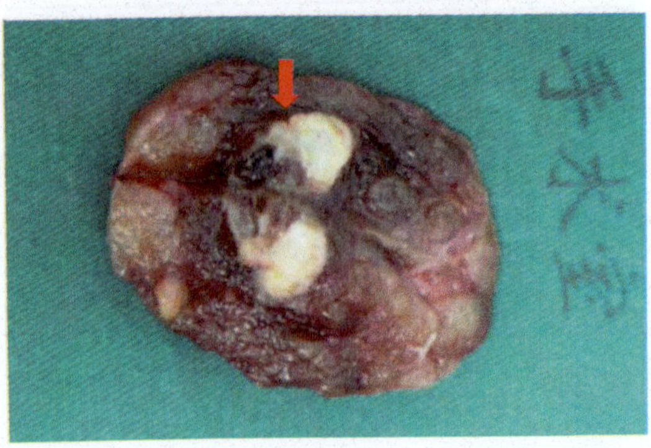

Fig. 7.69 Gross specimen of Case 45. A gray-white nodule 1.1 cm in size was seen in the 0.5-cm distance from capsule

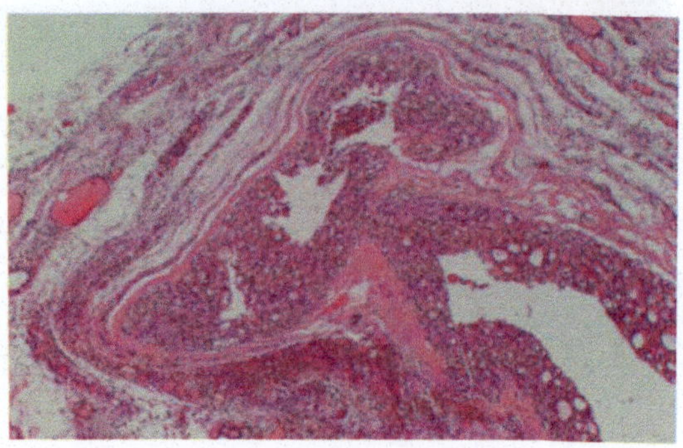

Fig. 7.70 Pathological diagnosis of Case 44 Atypical adenoma

Sonographic findings:

Thyroid scan

Left lobe: 4.3 cm × 1.3 cm × 1.2 cm.

Right lobe: 5.0 cm × 2.0 cm × 1.4 cm.

Isthmus: anteroposterior diameter is 0.27 cm.

Size and shape of the thyroid gland were normal. The echogenicity of parenchyma was uneven.

A 0.42 cm × 0.55 cm hypoechoic nodule with ill-defined margin irregular shape was detected in the left lobe, and no blood flow sign was observed.

A 0.65 cm × 0.63 cm anechoic nodule with ill-defined margin and increased echogenicity behind was detected in the middle of right lobe. It was a cyst-solid mixed nodule with hyperechogenicity inside, and few blood flow sign was observed.

Sonographic indicates:

Hypoechoic nodule in the isthmus of thyroid (TI-RADS 4b)

Cyst-solid mixed nodule in the right lobe (TI-RADS 3)

Fig. 7.71 Sonographic report of Case 46

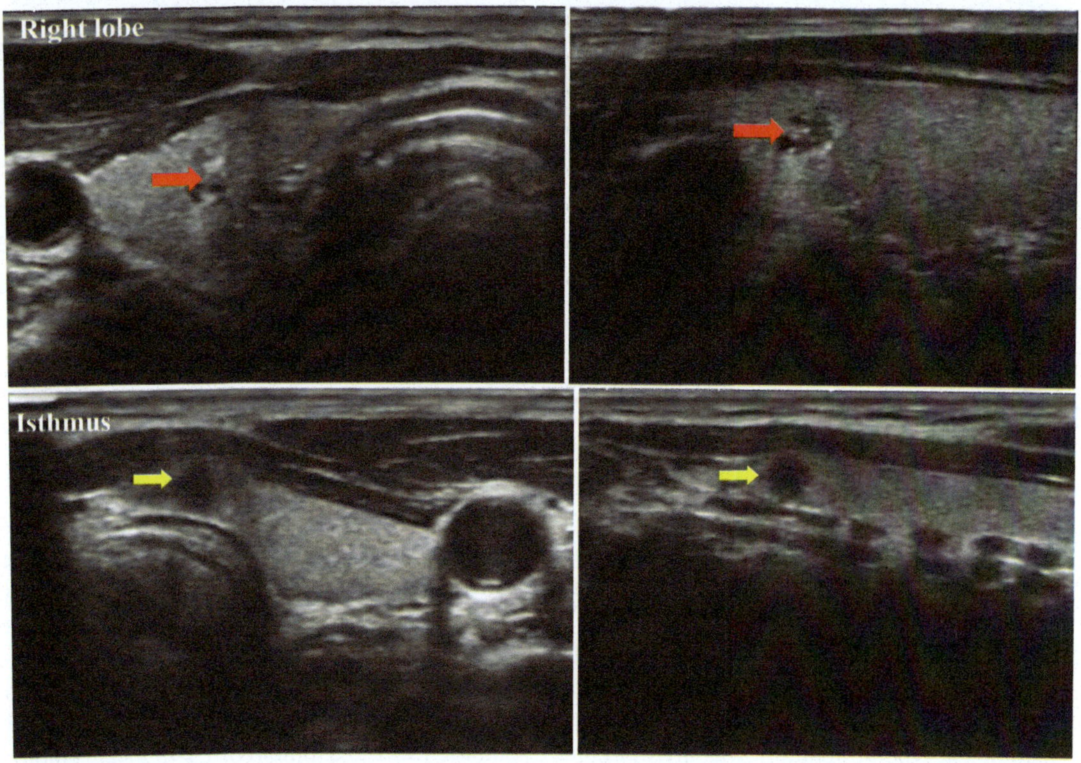

Fig. 7.72 Preoperative ultrasonic reevaluation of Case 46. Hyperechoic foci were observed in the right nodule, however, it was difficult to distinguish malignancy. mixed nodule in the right lobe. Fine needle aspiration cytology was recommended

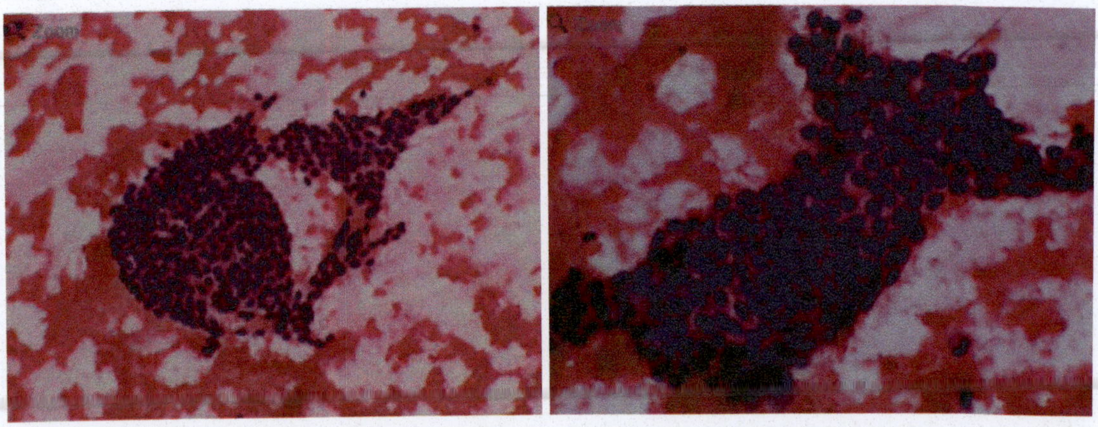

Fig. 7.73 Reports of fine needle aspiration cytology for Case 46. Papillary thyroid carcinoma. A large number of heterotypic follicular epithelial cells were observed microscopically, and the nuclear sulcus and nuclear overlap could be seen

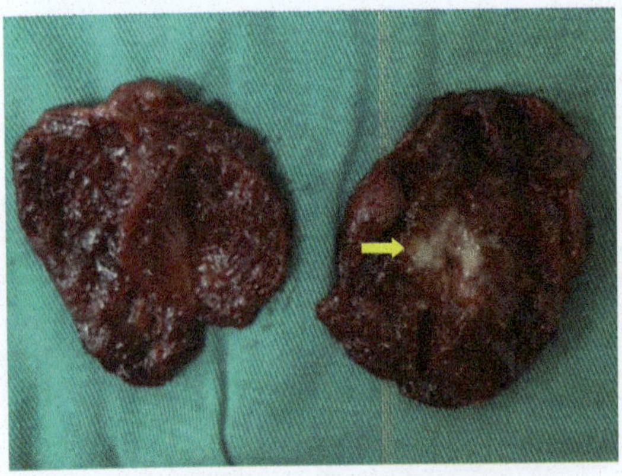

Fig. 7.74 Gross specimen of Case 45. A gray-white nodule 0.8 cm in size was observed

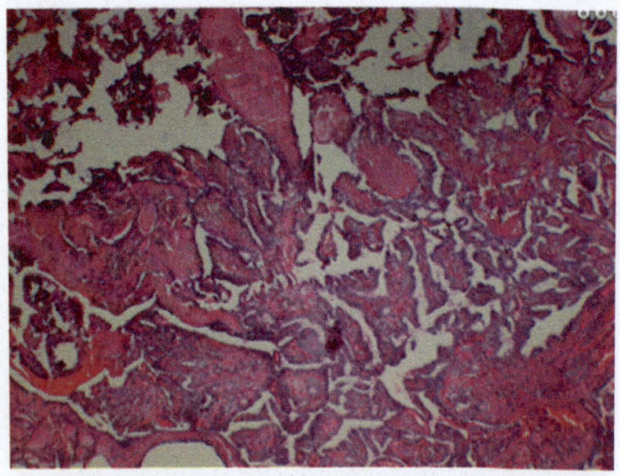

Fig. 7.75 Pathological diagnosis of Case 44 (left) Papillary thyroid carcinoma (right). Papillary thyroid microcarcinoma

eccentric obtuse shape, smooth free edge of solid part, no obvious blood flow or peripheral blood flow signal in nodules, spongy shape, and isoechogenicity in solid module.

Hypoechoic halo surrounded the nodule 2. Hypoechoic halo is a low or anechoic ring surrounding a nodule, composed of fibrous connective tissues, compressed thyroid tissues, or chronic inflammatory infiltrated tissues, can also be a vascular structure (Fig. 7.82).

Gross specimen and pathological diagnosis: Histological type of nodule 1 was thyroid goiter with hemorrhagic cystic degeneration, nodule 2 was nodular thyroid goiter (Figs. 7.83 and 7.84).

Case 49

Clinical information: A 45-year-old female patient was detected with thyroid nodule for half a year. Specialized physical examination: A tough nodule about 1.0 cm in the right thyroid lobe could be palpated, which moves up and down along with swallowing. FT3: 4.43 pmol/L (3.21–6.5 pmol/L), FT4: 17.25 pmol/L

Ultrasonic images:

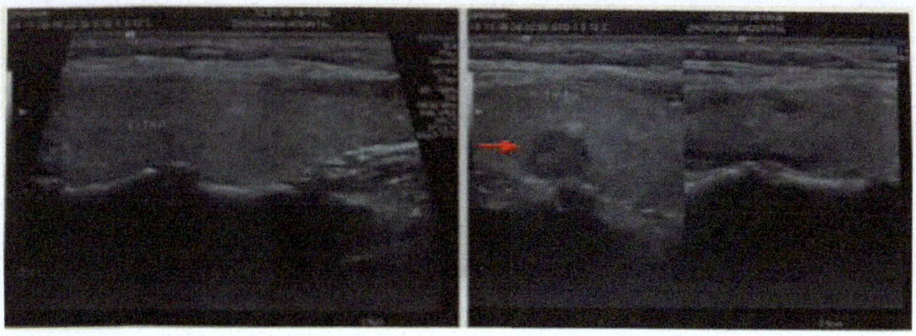

Sonographic findings:

Thyroid scan

Left lobe: 4.8 cm × 1.7 cm× 1.4 cm.

Right lobe: 4.6 cm × 1.7 cm× 1.2 cm.

Isthmus: anteroposterior diameter is 0.25 cm.

Size and shape of the thyroid gland were normal.

Two hypoechoic nodules with clear margin and uneven echogenicity inside was detected in the superior of the right lobe. The nodules were 0.8 cm × 0.6 cm, 0.5 cm × 0.2 cm in size, the larger contained hyperechogenicity inside.

CDFI: Few blood flow sign was observed.

Sonographic indicates:

Hypoechoic nodule in the right lobe (TI-RADS 3)

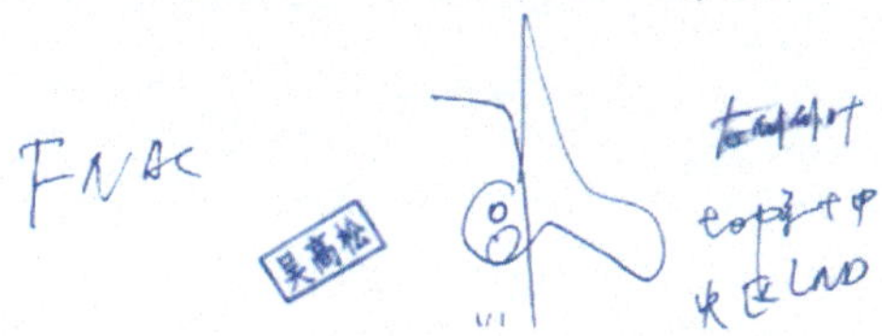

Fig. 7.76 Sonographic report of Case 47

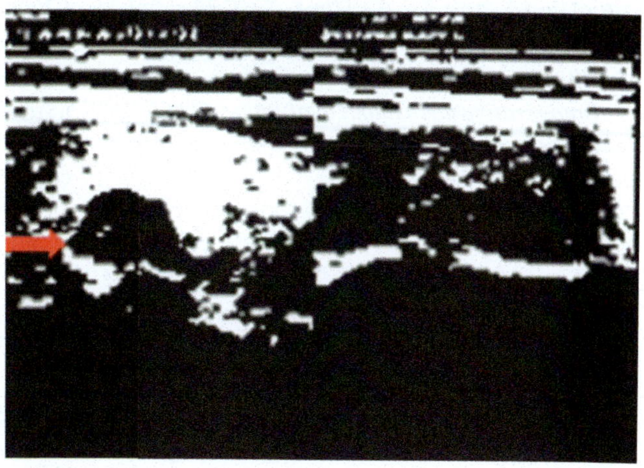

Fig. 7.77 Processed sonographic report of Case 47. After the image is processed, false foot on the edge of the nodule could be observed

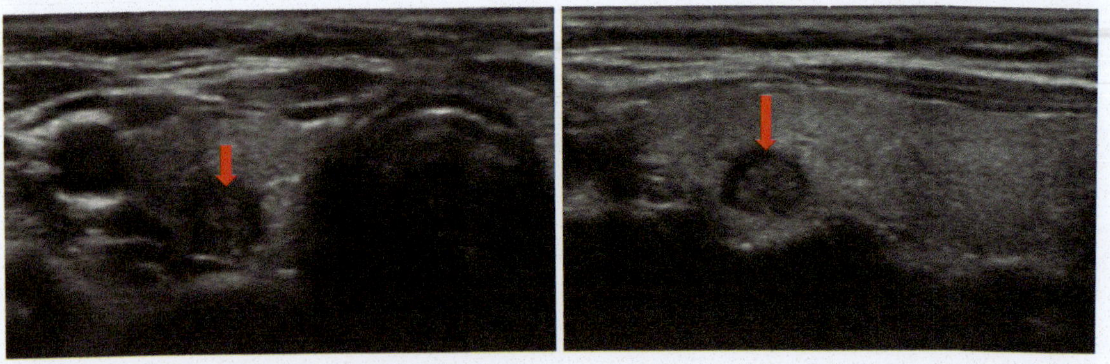

Fig. 7.78 Preoperative ultrasonic reevaluation of Case 47

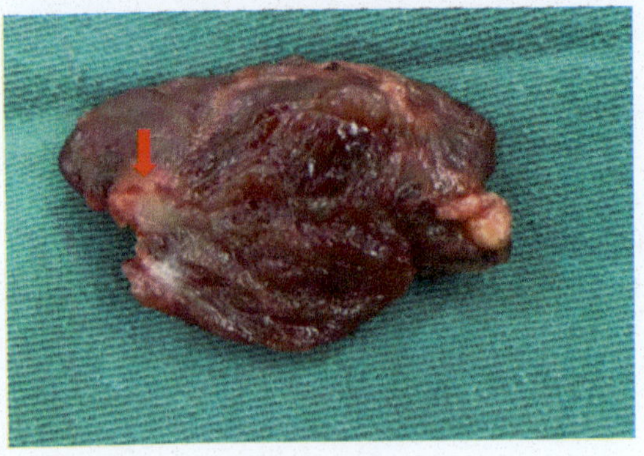

Fig. 7.79 Gross specimen of Case 45. A gray-white nodule 0.7 cm in size was observed at 0.1 cm distance from capsule

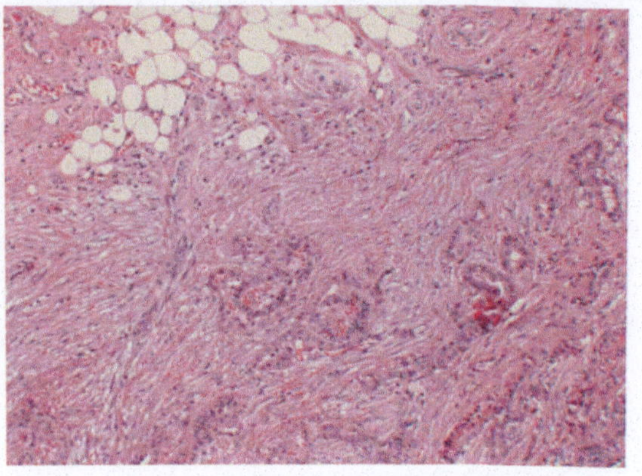

Fig. 7.80 Pathological diagnosis of Case 44 Papillary thyroid carcinoma, invading the capsule

(10.22–21.88 pmol/L), TSH: 3.04 μU/mL (0.3–4.6 μU/mL), Anti-Tg: 83 U/mL ↑ (0–72 U/mL), A-TPO: 80 U/mL ↑ (0–16 U/mL).

Ultrasonic information: Fig. 7.85.

Preoperative ultrasound evaluation: Fig. 7.86.

Gross specimen and pathological diagnosis: Figs. 7.87 and 7.88.

Case 50

Clinical information: A 29-year-old female patient was detected with thyroid nodules for one year. T3, T4, and TSH levels were normal.

Ultrasonic information: Fig. 7.89.

Preoperative ultrasound evaluation: Fig. 7.90.

Gross specimen and pathological diagnosis: Figs. 7.91 and 7.92.

Case 51

Clinical information: A 55-year-old female patient was detected with bilateral thyroid nodules for two years. T3, T4, and TSH levels were normal. Specialized physical examination: A tough nodule about 2.0 cm in the left thyroid lobe could be palpated, which moves up and down along with swallowing.

Ultrasonic information: Figs. 7.83 and 7.93.

Preoperative ultrasound evaluation: Fig. 7.94.

Gross specimen and pathological diagnosis: Figs. 7.91 and 7.95.

Case 52

Clinical information: A 46-year-old male patient was detected with thyroid nodule for half a year.

Ultrasonic images:

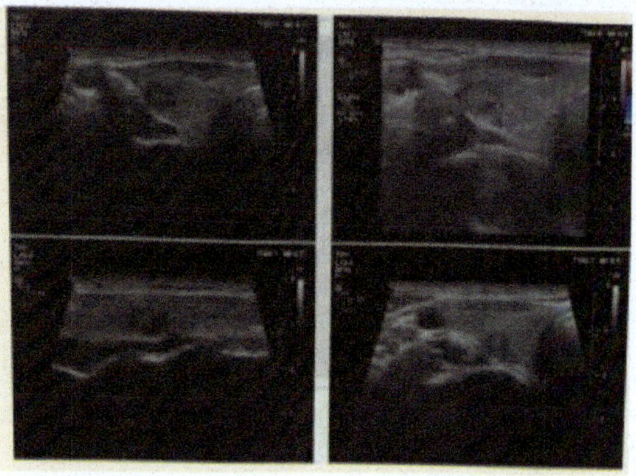

Sonographic findings:

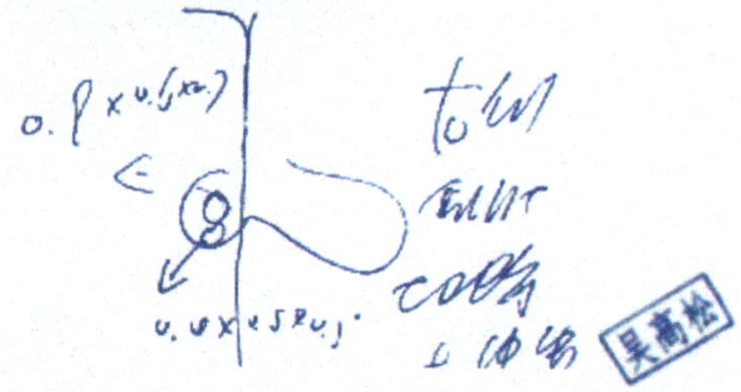

Thyroid scan

Left lobe: 4.2 cm × 1.8 cm × 1.2 cm.

Right lobe: 5.8 cm × 1.9 cm × 1.1 cm.

Isthmus: anteroposterior diameter is 0.24 cm.

Size and shape of the thyroid gland were normal. The echogenicity of parenchyma was uneven.

A 0.9 cm × 0.6 cm × 0.7 cm hypoechoic nodule with clear margin and uneven echogenicity was detected in the right lobe. Punctate hyperechogenicity was detected in the nodule and no blood flow sign was observed.

A taller than wide 0.4 cm × 0.5 cm × 0.5 cm hypoechoic nodule with ill-defined margin and uneven echogenicity was detected in the right lobe. No blood flow sign was observed.

Sonographic indicates:

Hypoechoic nodule with calcification in the right lobe (TI-RADS 4b)

Taller than wide hypoechoic nodule with calcification in the right lobe (TI-RADS 4a)

Fig. 7.81 Sonographic report of Case 48

Specialized physical examination: A tough nodule about 2.5 cm in the left thyroid lobe could be palpated, which moves up and down along with swallowing. FT3: 5.13 pmol/L (3.21–6.5 pmol/L) FT4: 16.34 pmol/L (10.22–21.88 pmol/L), TSH: 2.64 μU/mL (0.3–4.6 μU/mL), Anti-Tg: 14 U/mL (0–72 U/mL), A-TPO 55 U/mL ↑ (0–16 U/mL), calcitonin: 1190 pg/mL (18 pg/mL).

Ultrasonic information: Ultrasound at the time of outpatient visit TI-RADS class 5, the patient has elevated calcitonin, so total thyroid resection is recommended. Postoperative pathological examination results show left medullary thyroid cancer. Medullary thyroid carcinoma (medullary thyroid carcinoma, MTC), clinically rare, lymph node metastasis early, high degree

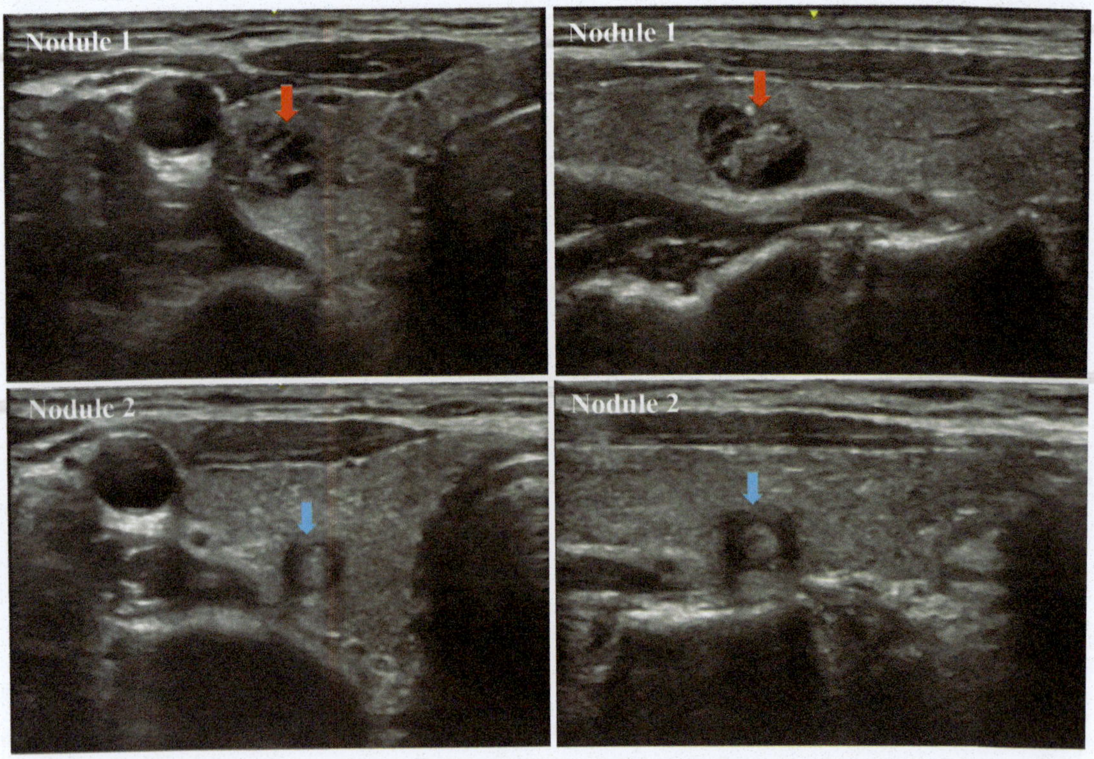

Fig. 7.82 Preoperative ultrasonic reevaluation of Case 47. Nodule 1: hypoechoic nodule with calcification in the right lobe (TI-RADS 4b). Nodule 2: taller than wide hypoechoic nodule with calcification in the right lobe (TI-RADS 4a)

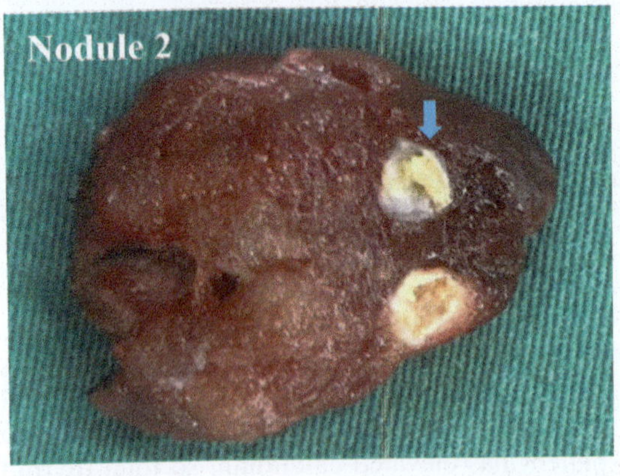

Fig. 7.83 Gross specimen of Case 48. A gray-white nodule 0.4 cm in size was observed at 0.1 cm distance from capsule

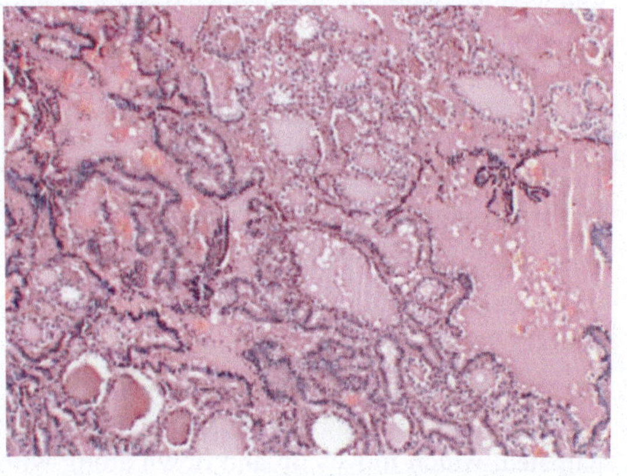

Fig. 7.84 Pathological diagnosis of Case 48 (nodule 2) Nodular goiter with bleeding cystic degeneration

Ultrasonic images:

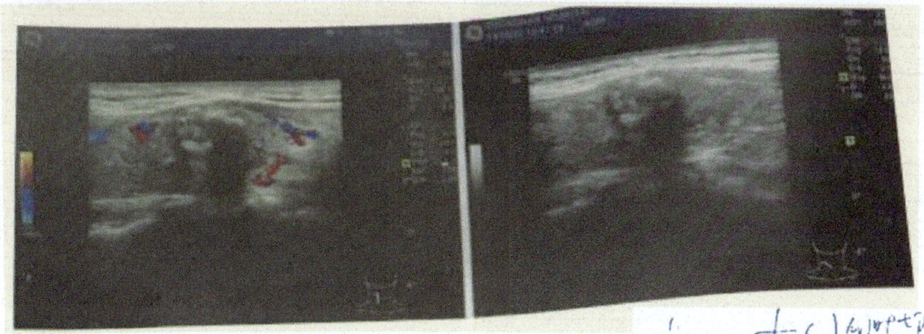

Sonographic findings:

Isthmus: anteroposterior diameter is 0.23 cm.

Size and shape of the thyroid gland were normal. The echogenic hypoechoic and uneven. Two hypoechoic nodules with clear ma ity inside was detected in the right lobe. The nodules were 1.4 cm × 1.1 cm, 0.9 cm × 0.5 cm in size with hyperechogenicity inside.

CDFI: Few blood flow sign was observed

Sonographic indicates:

Diffuse lesions of the thyroid gland
Hypoechoic nodule with calcification in the right lobe (TI-RADS 3)

Fig. 7.85 Sonographic report of Case 49

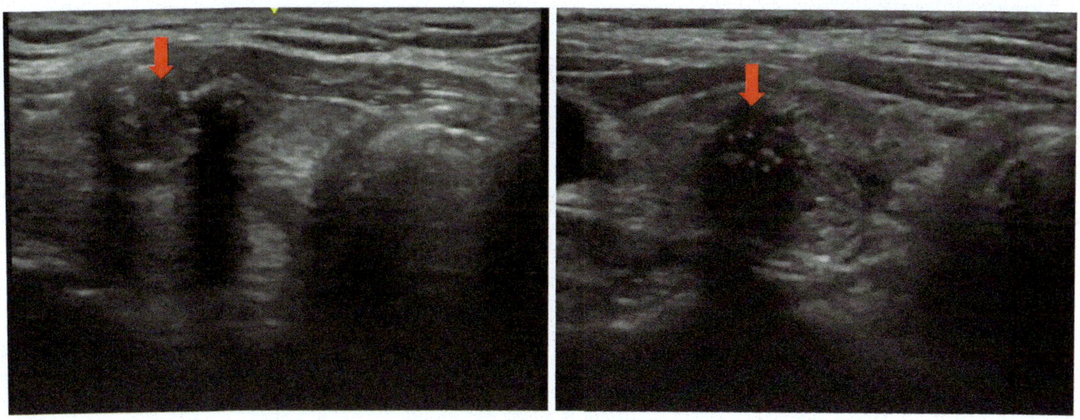

Fig. 7.86 Preoperative ultrasonic reevaluation of Case 49. Irregular hypoechoic nodule with punctate hyperechogenicity inside in the right lobe

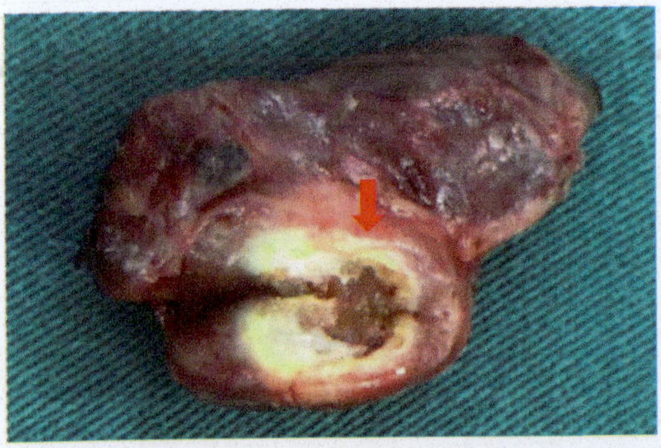

Fig. 7.87 Gross specimen of Case 49. A gray white hard nodule 1.4 cm in size close to capsule was observed

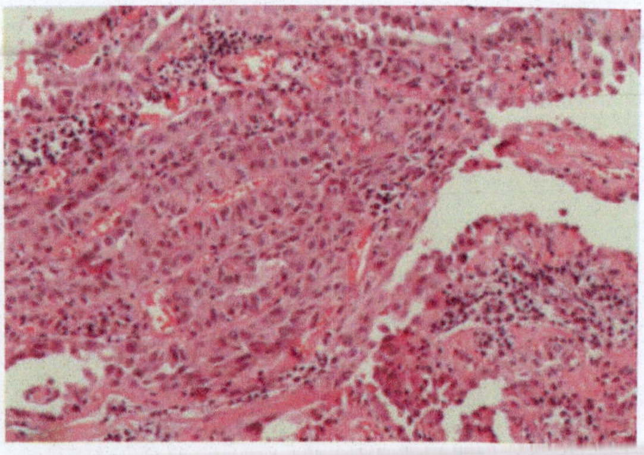

Fig. 7.88 Pathological diagnosis of Case 48. Papillary thyroid carcinoma

Ultrasonic images:

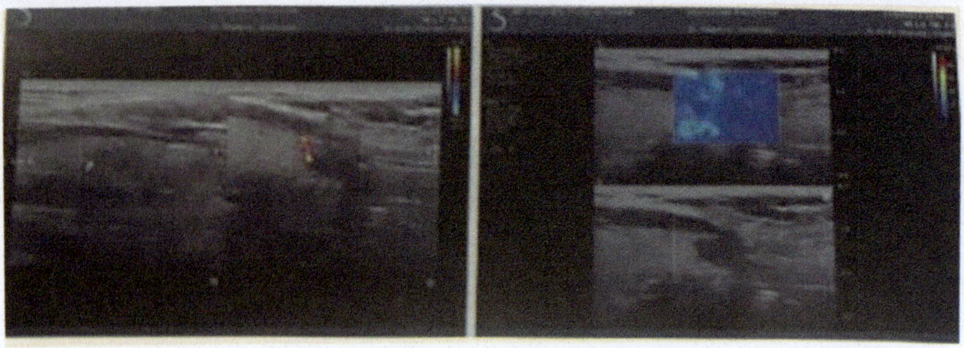

Sonographic findings:

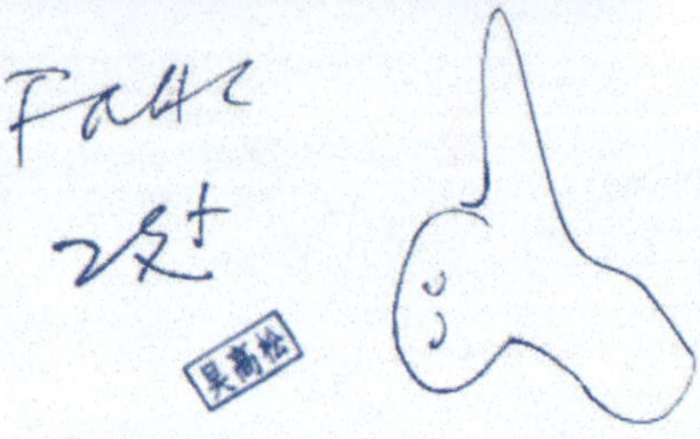

Thyroid scan

Left lobe: 4.2 cm × 1.5 cm × 1.3 cm.

Right lobe: 4.6 cm × 1.5 cm × 1.4 cm.

Isthmus: anteroposterior diameter is 0.37 cm.

The echogenicity of parenchyma was uneven. Two hypoechoic nodules with clear margin and uniform echogenicity inside was detected in the inferior of right lobe. The nodules were 0.8 cm × 0.5 cm, 0.8 cm × 0.6 cm in size with blood flow signs.

Sonographic indicates:

Solid nodule in the right lobe (adenoma? TI-RADS 3)

Fig. 7.89 Sonographic report of Case 50

of malignancy, poor prognosis, common ultrasound manifestations of medullary thyroid carcinoma, including MTC cancer cells are large and overlapping, low degree of differentiation, good tumor sound transmittance, ultrasound often presents low echo; the side boundary of MTC is not as clear as follicular thyroid adenoma (FTA). However, it is clearer than papillary thyroid carcinoma (PTC); the surrounding halo of MTC is a low echo, incomplete or uneven in thickness, the surrounding halo of FTA is echoless and relatively complete; the blood flow inside MTC is abundant and the walking is disordered; calcification is visible in half of the lesions of MTC, mainly microcalcification (Figs. 7.96 and 7.97).

Case 53

Clinical information: A 40-year-old female patient was detected with left thyroid nodules for one month. FT3: 5.56 pmol/L (3.21–6.5pmol/L), FT4: 13.38 pmol/L (10.22–21.88 pmol/L), TSH: 3.39 μU/mL (0.3–4.6 μU/mL), Anti-Tg: 81 U/mL ↑(0–72 U/mL), A-TPO 545 U/mL ↑(0–16 U/mL)

Ultrasonic information: Fig. 7.98.

Preoperative ultrasound evaluation: Fig. 7.99.

Gross specimen and pathological diagnosis: Figs. 7.100 and 7.101.

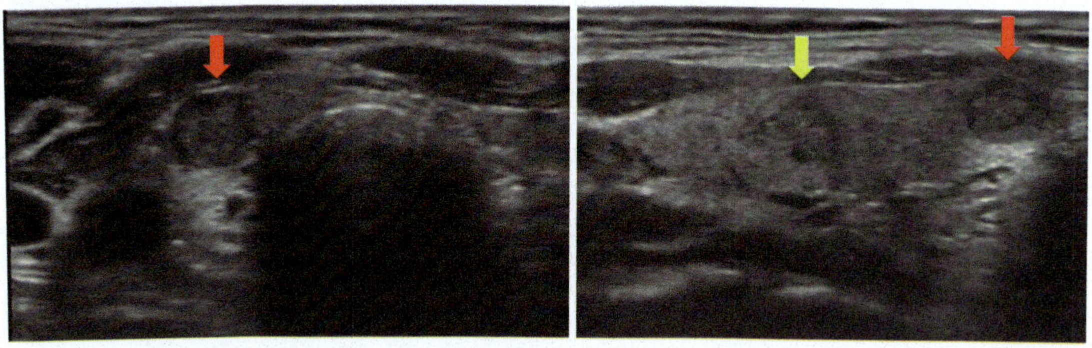

Fig. 7.90 Preoperative ultrasonic reevaluation of Case 50

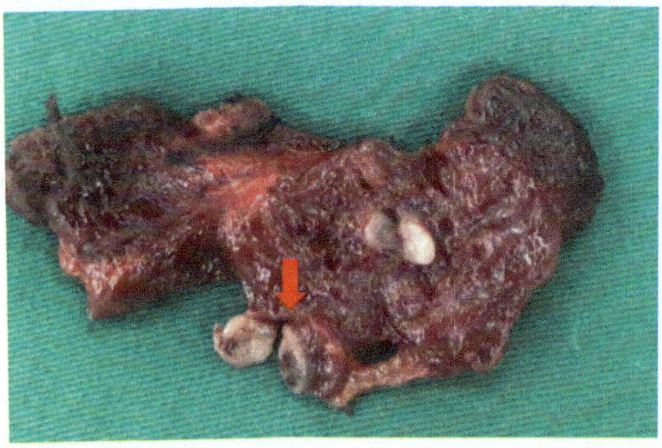

Fig. 7.91 Gross specimen of Case 49. A gray-white hard nodule 1.4 cm in size close to capsule was observed

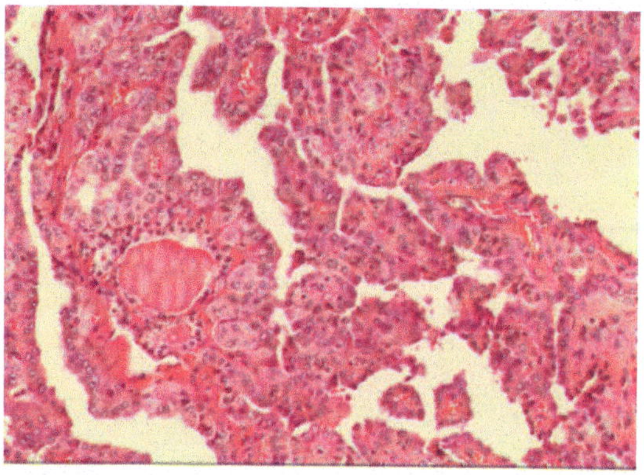

Fig. 7.92 Pathological diagnosis of Case 48. Papillary thyroid carcinoma

Ultrasonic images:

Thyroid scan

Size and shape of the thyroid gland were normal. The echogenicity of parenchyma was uneven.

Two anechoic nodules with clear margin and increased echogenicity behind were detected in the left lobe, one of which was 1.2 cm × 1.5 cm in size, and no blood flow sign was observed.

Several hypoechoic areas with ill-defined margin and irregular shape were observed in the right lobe and thyroid isthmus, one of which was 4.3 cm × 0.9 cm in size, and blood flow sign was observed. A sightly low hypoechoic 2.1 cm × 1.5 cm nodule with clear margin and uneven echogenicity inside was observed in the right lobe, in which a 0.35 cm × 0.05 cm hyperechoic foci was seen with acoustic shadowing behind, and blood flow sign was observed.

Sonographic indicates:

Cystic nodule in the left lobe (TI-RADS 2)

Hyperechoic nodule in the right lobe and isthmus of thyroid (TI-RADS 4a)

Hyperechoic nodule in the left lobe (TI-RADS 3)

Fig. 7.93 Sonographic report of Case 51

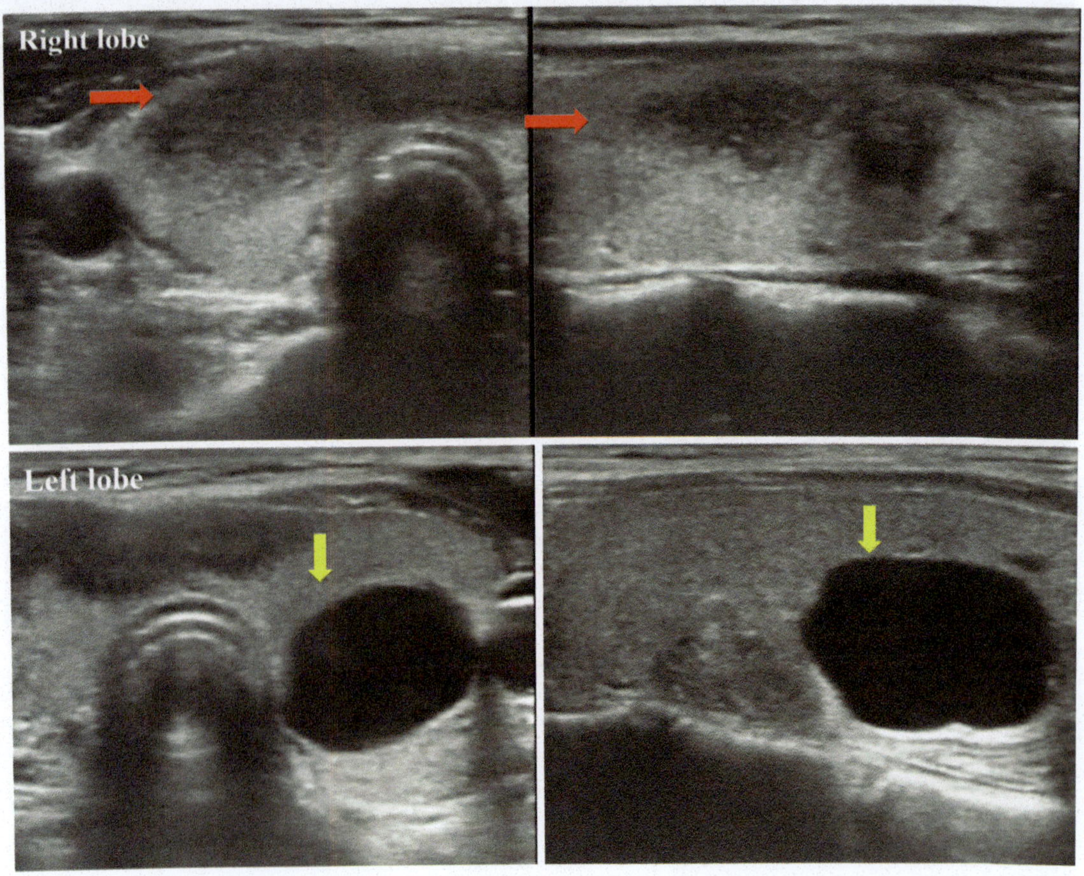

Fig. 7.94 Preoperative ultrasonic reevaluation of Case 51

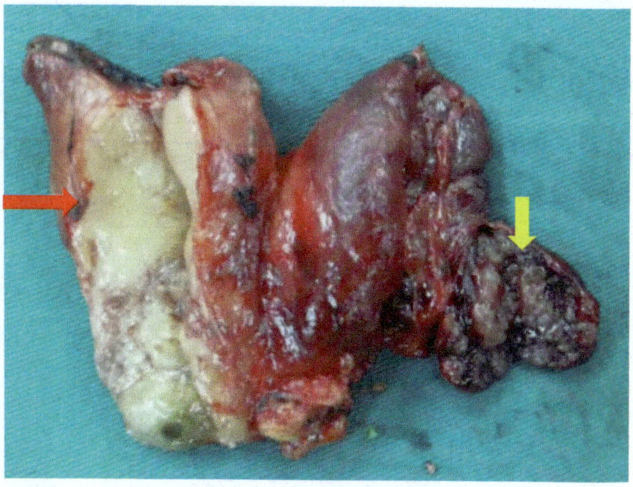

Fig. 7.95 Pathological diagnosis of Case 48. A 2 cm× 1.5 cm× 1 cm reddish-brown cyst-solid nodule in the left lobe. A 4 cm× 2.5 cm× 1.5 cm gray-yellow irregular lesion area with calcification in right lobe. A 2 cm cystic solid jelly-like nodule close to the gray-yellow lesion area in the inferior pole of right lobe. Histological type: Bilateral papillary thyroid carcinoma

Ultrasonic images:

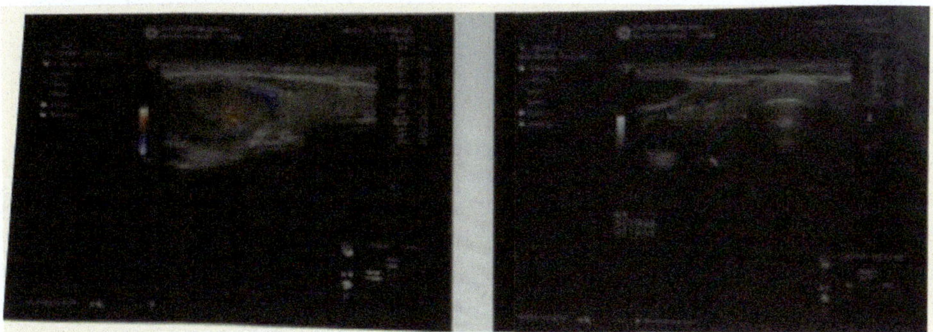

Sonographic findings:

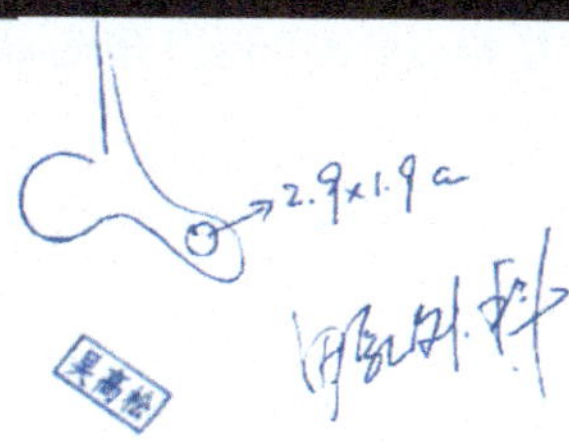

Thyroid scan

Left lobe: 2.2 cm × 1.8 cm.

Right lobe: 1.7 cm × 1.3 cm.

Isthmus: anteroposterior diameter is 0.2 cm. The echogenicity of parenchyma was uniform.

An oval wide than taller 2.9 cm × 1.9 cm hypoechoic nodule with clear margin and uneven echogenicity inside was detected in the left lobe. Punctate echogenicity and blood flow signs were observed in this nodule.

CDFI: Blood flow signs of the thyroid did not significantly increase.

Sonographic indicates:

Solid nodule with calcification in the left lobe (TI-RADS 4a)

Fig. 7.96 Sonographic report of Case 52 (1)

Ultrasonic images:

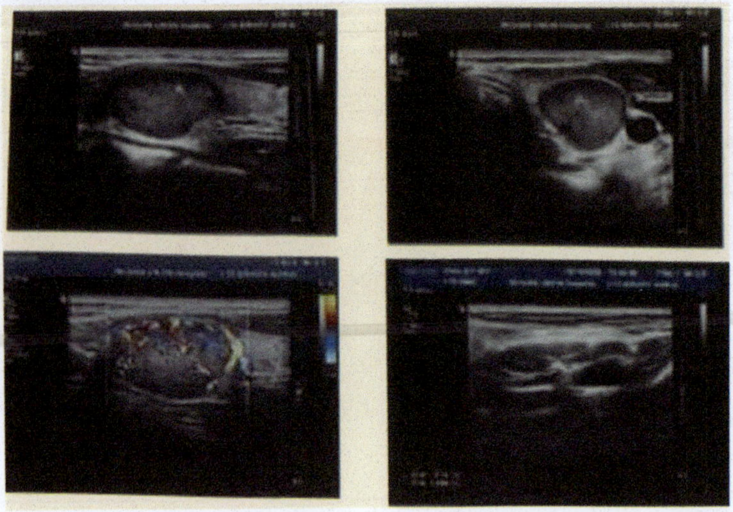

Sonographic findings:

Thyroid scan:

Shape of the right lobe and isthmus of the thyroid was normal, shape of the left lobe was sightly plump. A 29.5 mm × 22.2 mm × 19.1 mm hypoechoic solid nodule with clear margin was detected in the middle superior of left lobe. It was a wide than taller nodule with several punctate hyperechogenicity inside.

CDFI: Abundant blood flow signs were observed in the left hypoechoic nodule.

Several lymphatic echogenicity were observed in the bilateral neck with clear margin, two of them were 21.4 mm × 7.0 mm and 17.8 mm × 6.4 mm in left and right level II

CDFI: No blood flow was observed in the lymph nodes.

Sonographic indicates:

Solid nodule with calcification in the left lobe (TI-RADS 4a)

Lymph nodes in the bilateral neck

Fig. 7.97 Sonographic report of Case 52 (2)

Ultrasonic images:

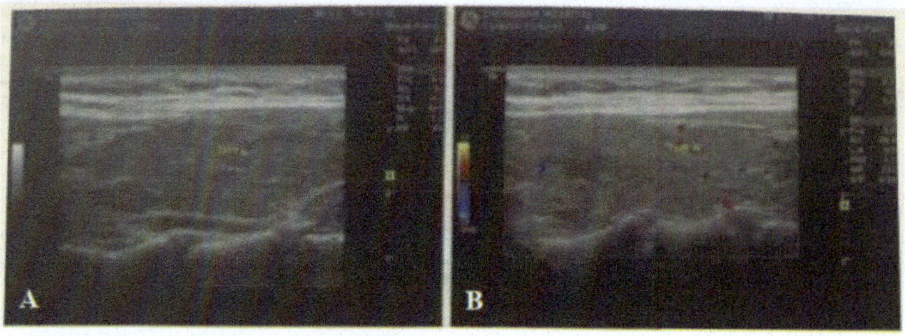

Sonographic findings:

Thyroid scan

Left lobe: 5.0 cm × 1.7 cm × 1.4 cm.

Right lobe: 5.0 cm × 1.8 cm × 1.6 cm.

Isthmus: anteroposterior diameter is 0.32 cm.

The echogenicity of parenchyma was sightly decreased and uneven. A 1.0 cm × 0.6 cm hypoechoic nodule with ill-defined margin and uneven echogenicity inside was detected in the inferior of left lobe (A). A 0.9 cm × 0.6 cm sightly low hypoechoic nodule with ill-defined margin and uneven echogenicity inside was detected in the inferior of right lobe (B).

Sonographic indicates:

Diffuse lesions of the thyroid gland

Hypoechoic nodule in the left lobe (TI-RADS 4a)

Sightly low hypoechoic nodule in the right lobe (TI-RADS 3)

Fig. 7.98 Sonographic report of Case 53

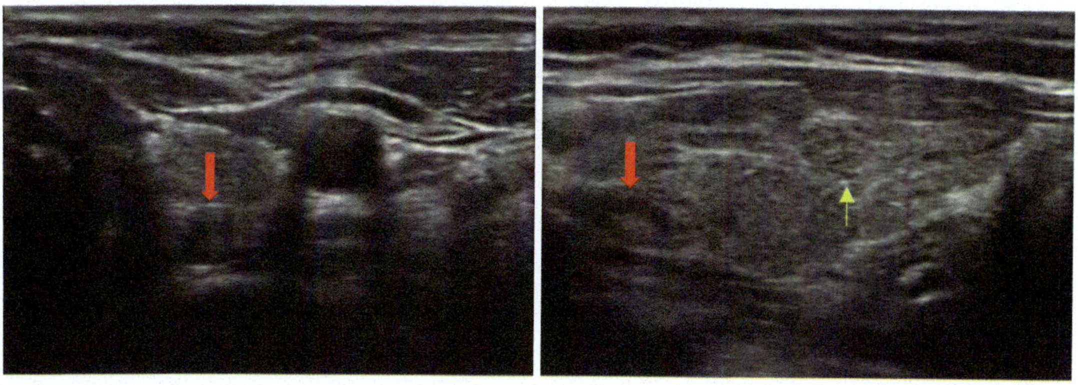

Fig. 7.99 Preoperative ultrasonic reevaluation of Case 53. Decreased echogenicity in the thyroid gland, short line hyperechogenicity formed by fibrous hyperplasia (yellow arrow)

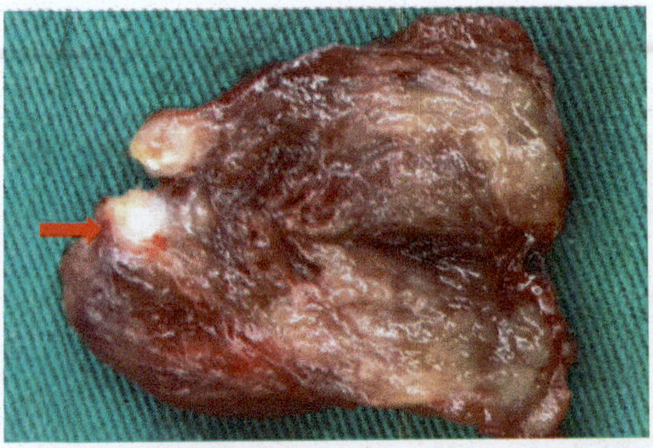

Fig. 7.100 Gross specimen of Case 53. A gray-white-gray-yellow nodule

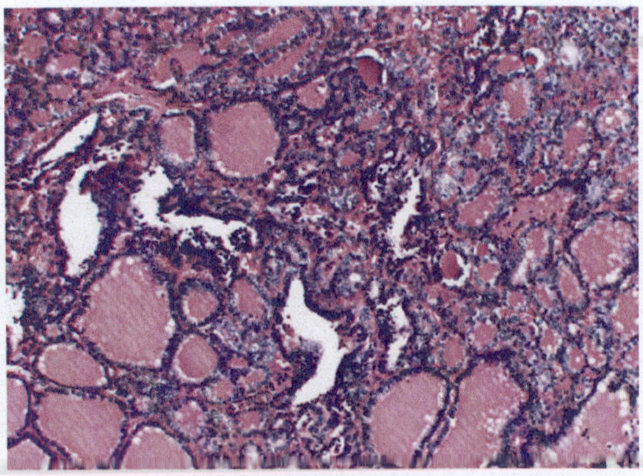

Fig. 7.101 Pathological diagnosis of Case 53. Left thyroiditis, local fibrosis formation

Ultrasonic images:

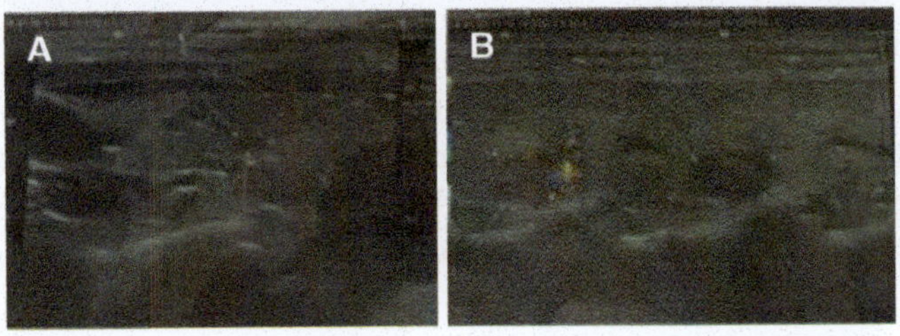

Sonographic findings:

Thyroid scan

Shape of the thyroid was normal. The echogenicity of parenchyma was uneven. A 1.0 cm × 0.6 cm hypoechoic nodule with clear margin was detected in the middle inferior of right lobe, no blood flow was detected (A). A 0.78 cm × 0.56 cm hypoechoic solid nodule with clear margin was detected in the middle superior of left lobe, and blood flow was detected (B).

Sonographic indicates:

Hypoechoic nodule in the middle inferior of right lobe (TI-RADS 3)

Hypoechoic solid nodule in the middle superior of left lobe (TI-RADS 4a)

Fig. 7.102 Sonographic report of Case 54 (01/2018)

Case 54

Clinical information: A 45-year-old male patient was detected with thyroid nodule for one year. Specialized physical examination: A tough nodule about 0.5 cm × 0.4 cm in the left thyroid lobe could be palpated, which moves up and down along with swallowing. FT3: 4.53pmol/L (3.21–6.5 pmol/L), FT4: 13.64 pmol/L (10.22–21.88 pmol/L), TSH: 2.19 μU/mL (0.3–4.6 μU/mL), Anti-Tg 468 U/mL ↑ (0–72 U/mL), A-TPO: 29 U/mL ↑ (0–16 U/mL).

Ultrasonic information: Figs. 7.102, 7.103, and 7.104

Preoperative ultrasound evaluation: Fig. 7.105.

Ultrasonic images:

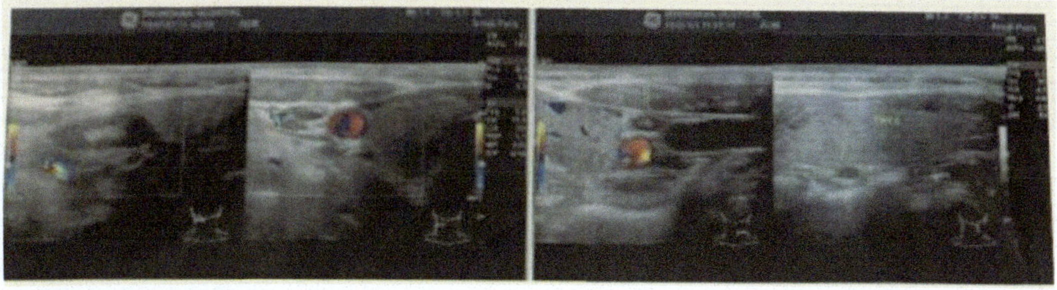

Sonographic findings:

Bilateral neck scan:

Right:

Several hypoechoic masses with lymphatic hilum and clear cortex and medulla was detected in level II of right neck, one of which was 1.9 cm × 0.7 cm in size.

Several hypoechoic masses with lymphatic hilum and clear cortex and medulla was detected in level III of right neck, one of which was 0.8 cm × 0.3 cm in size.

Left:

Several hypoechoic masses with lymphatic hilum and clear cortex and medulla was detected in level II of left neck, one of which was 1.2 cm × 0.8 cm in size.

Several hypoechoic masses with lymphatic hilum and clear cortex and medulla was detected in level III of left neck, one of which was 0.6 cm × 0.4 cm in size.

CDFI: Colored blood flow signals are not visible in the above hypoechoic masses.

A 0.44 cm × 0.30 cm hypoechoic nodule with clear margin was detected in the dorsal superior of left lobe, and no blood flow was detected.

Sonographic indicates:

Bilateral cervical lymph nodes were detected

Hypoechoic nodule in the dorsal superior of left lobe (parathyroid gland? central neck lymph node?)

Fig. 7.103 Sonographic report of Case 54 (07/2019)

Gross specimen and pathological diagnosis: Figs. 7.106 and 7.107.

Case 55

Clinical information: A 62-year-old female patient was detected with thyroid nodule for half a month. FT3: 4.83 pmol/L (3.21–6.5 pmol/L), FT4: 12.43 pmol/L (10.22–21.88 pmol/L), TSH: 5.05 µU/mL (0.3–4.6 µU/mL), Anti-Tg: 12 U/mL (0–72 U/mL), A-TPO: 7 U/mL (0–16 U/mL).

Ultrasonic information: Fig. 7.108.

Preoperative ultrasound evaluation: Fig. 7.109.

Gross specimen and pathological diagnosis: Figs. 7.110 and 7.111.

Ultrasonic images:

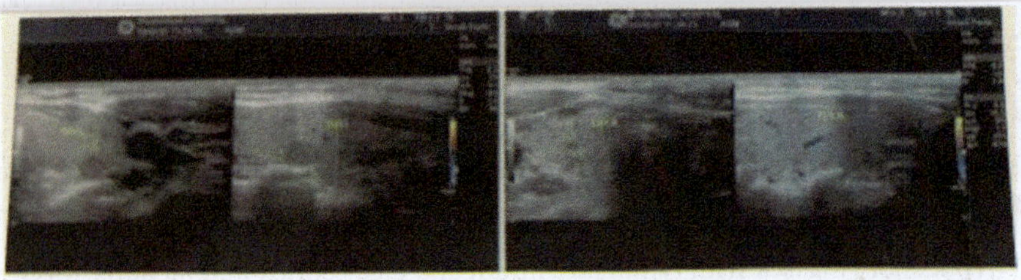

Sonographic findings:

Thyroid scan

Shape of the thyroid was normal. The echogenicity of parenchyma was sightly low and uneven with patchy hypoechogenicity inside. A taller than wide 0.67 cm × 0.56 cm × 0.55 cm hypoechoic nodule with clear margin was detected in the left lobe. A 0.24 cm × 0.19 cm sightly low hypoechoic nodule with clear margin was detected in the right lobe.

CDFI: Few blood flow signs were detected in the left hypoechoic nodule, no blood flow sign was observed in the right sightly low hypoechoic nodule.

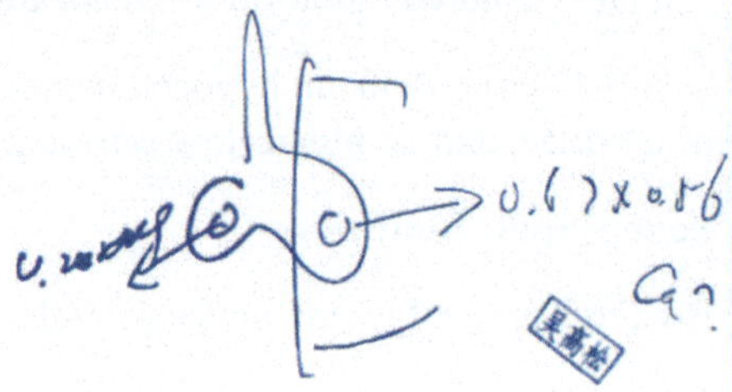

Sonographic indicates:

Diffuse lesions of the thyroid gland

Hypoechoic nodule in the left lobe (TI-RADS 4b)

Sightly low hypoechoic solid nodule in the right lobe (TI-RADS 3)

Fig. 7.104 Sonographic report of Case 54 (10/2019)

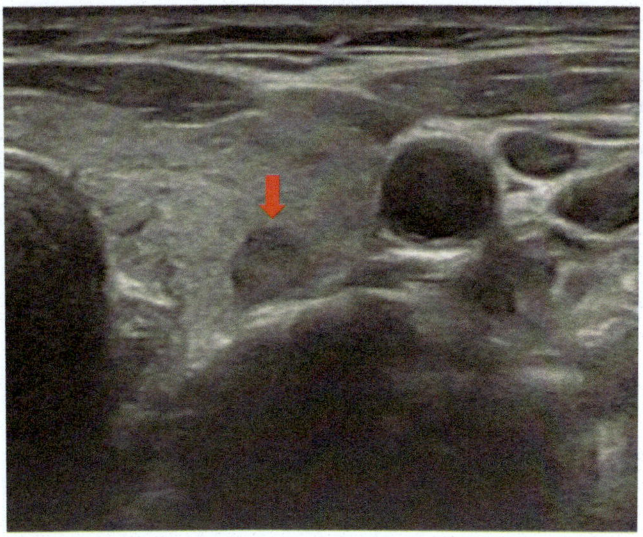

Scan the QR code
to watch the ultrasonic video

Fig. 7.105 Preoperative ultrasonic reevaluation of Case 54

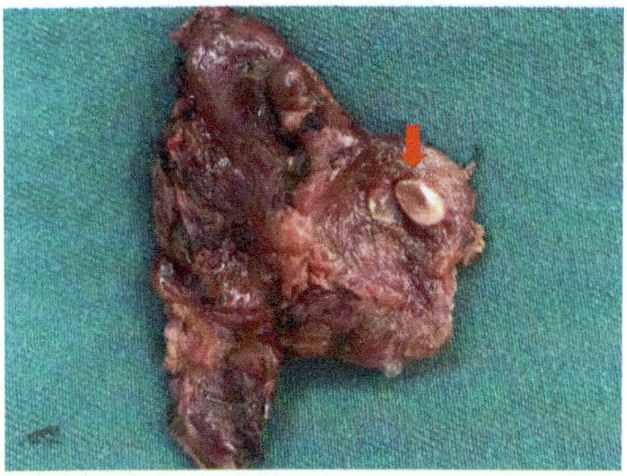

Fig. 7.106 Gross specimen of Case 54. A 0.7-cm gray-white nodule with a soft texture

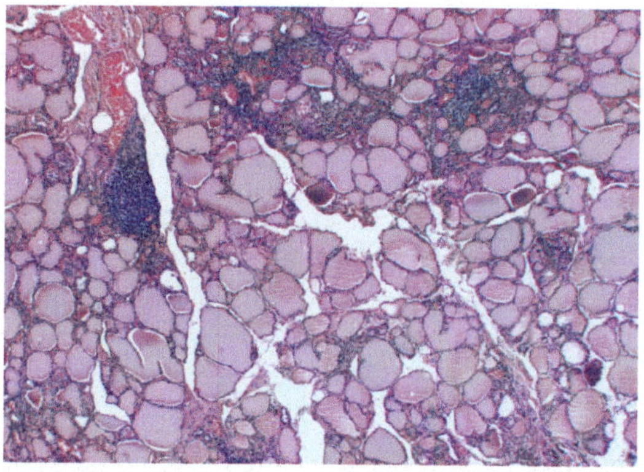

Fig. 7.107 Pathological diagnosis of Case 53. Nodular thyroid goiter concomitant with lymph node hyperplasia and local fibrosis, vitreous changes

Ultrasonic images:

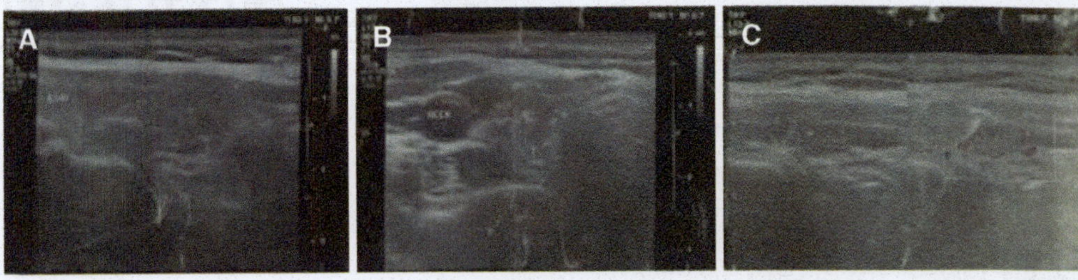

Sonographic findings:

Thyroid scan

Left lobe: 3.2 cm × 1.0 cm × 0.9 cm.

Right lobe: 3.6 cm × 1.1 cm × 1.1 cm.

Isthmus: anteroposterior diameter is 0.20 cm.

Shape of the thyroid was normal. The echogenicity of parenchyma was uneven.

A 1.2 cm × 0.8 cm × 1.0 cm sightly low hypoechoic nodule with ill-defined margin and uneven echogenicity inside was detected in the inferior of right lobe, and punctate hyperechogenicity was observed (A and B).

CDFI: Few blood flow signs were detected in the right hypoechoic nodule,

A 0.7 cm × 0.4 cm sightly low hypoechoic nodule with ill-defined margin and uneven echogenicity inside was detected in the inferior of left lobe (C), and scutellate anechoic areas and short-line and fiber light band-like sightly high hyperechogenicity were observed with abundant blood flow signs.

Sonographic indicates:

Sightly low hypoechoic nodule with hyperechoic foci in the inferior of right lobe (TI-RADS 4b)

Sightly low hypoechoic nodule in the inferior of left lobe

Fig. 7.108 Sonographic report of Case 55

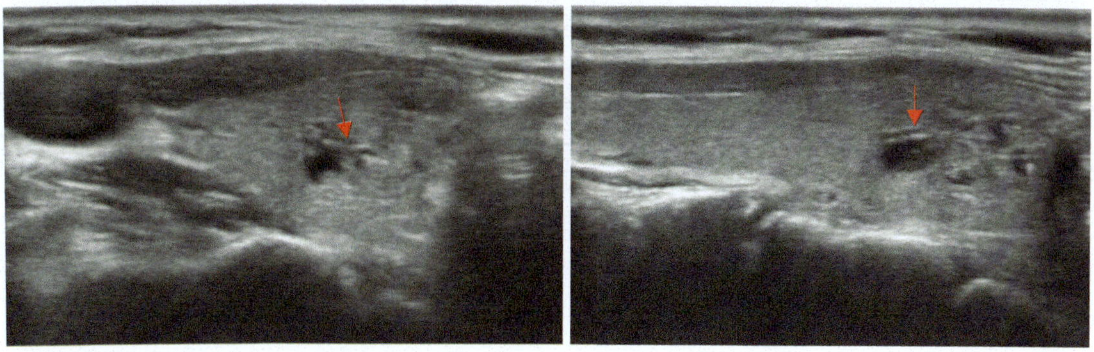

Fig. 7.109 Preoperative ultrasonic reevaluation of Case 55. Striped hyperechogenicity in the right nodule was easy to be diagnosed as punctate hyperechogenicity

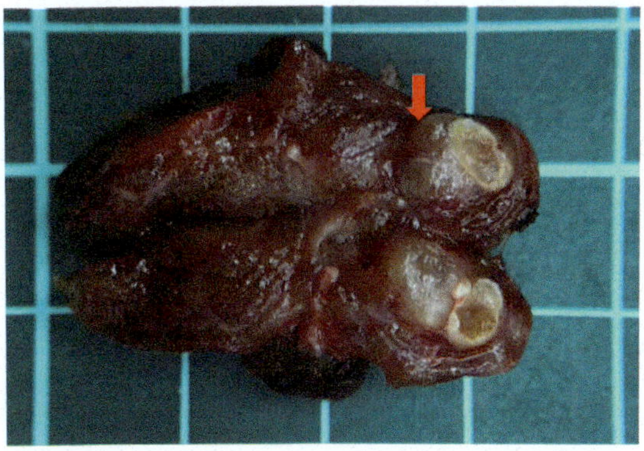

Fig. 7.110 Gross specimen of Case 55. A gray-white nodule 0.5 cm in size was observed at 0.2 cm distance from capsule

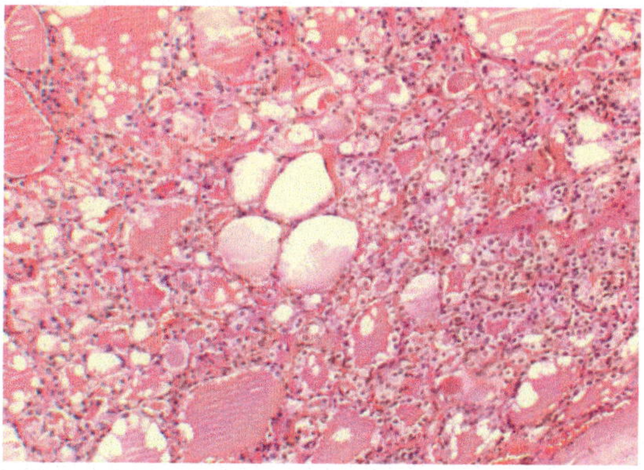

Fig. 7.111 Pathological diagnosis of Case 55 (right) Nodular thyroid goiter with adenoma nodules

The manufacturer's authorised representative in the EU is Springer Nature Customer Service Centre GmbH, Europaplatz 3, 69115 Heidelberg, Germany. If you have any concerns regarding our products, please contact ProductSafety@springernature.com

Printed and bound by CPI Group (UK) Ltd, Croydon, CR0 4YY
30/09/2026
02225266-0004